T0292260

The Pocket Guide to
Glaucoma

Ophthalmology Pocket Guides
Series

Series Editor, Richard L. Lindstrom

The Pocket Guide to
Glaucoma

EDITOR

Joseph F. Panarelli, MD
Associate Professor of Ophthalmology
Chief, Division of Glaucoma
Ophthalmology Department
New York University Langone Health
New York, New York

ASSOCIATE EDITORS

Davinder S. Grover, MD, MPH
Attending Surgeon and Clinician
Glaucoma Associates of Texas
Dallas, Texas

Arsham Sheybani, MD
Associate Professor
Residency Program Director
Glaucoma Fellowship Director
Washington University School of Medicine
St. Louis, Missouri

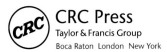

CRC Press
Taylor & Francis Group
Boca Raton London New York

CRC Press is an imprint of the
Taylor & Francis Group, an **informa** business

First published 2022 by SLACK Incorporated

Published 2024 by CRC Press
2385 NW Executive Center Drive, Suite 320, Boca Raton FL 33431

and by CRC Press
4 Park Square, Milton Park, Abingdon, Oxon, OX14 4RN

CRC Press is an imprint of Taylor & Francis Group, LLC

© 2022 Taylor & Francis Group, LLC

Cover Artist: Katherine Christie

Library of Congress Cataloging-in-Publication Data
Names: Panarelli, Joseph F., editor. | Grover, Davinder S., editor. |
  Sheybani, Arsham, editor.
Title: The pocket guide to glaucoma / editor, Joseph F. Panarelli ;
  associate editors, Davinder S. Grover, Arsham Sheybani.
Other titles: Glaucoma | Ophthalmology pocket guides.
Description: Thorofare, NJ : SLACK Incorporated, [2022] | Series:
  Ophthalmology pocket guides | Includes bibliographical references and
  index.
Identifiers: LCCN 2021048165 (print) | ISBN 9781630916701 (paperback)
Subjects: MESH: Glaucoma | Handbook | BISAC: MEDICAL / Ophthalmology |
  MEDICAL / Optometry
Classification: LCC RE871 (print) | NLM WW 39 | DDC
  617.7/41--dc23/eng/20211001
LC record available at https://lccn.loc.gov/2021048165

ISBN: 9781630916701 (pbk)
ISBN: 9781003525769 (ebk)

DOI: 10.1201/9781003525769

DEDICATION

To my wife, Nicole, and children, Joey and Nora. Thank you for the constant support and joy you bring to my life. You make each day more special than the last.

—*Joseph F. Panarelli, MD*

To my wife, my children, and my parents. Thank you for your constant love and support and for always inspiring me to be better, personally and professionally.

—*Davinder S. Grover, MD, MPH*

I dedicate this book to the educators that taught me how to teach and the families that supported them in life and work. Without a doubt, I could not do what I do without the support of my family and friends.

—*Arsham Sheybani, MD*

CONTENTS

ABOUT THE EDITOR

Joseph F. Panarelli, MD is an associate professor of ophthalmology at the New York University Grossman School of Medicine who specializes in the treatment of adult and pediatric glaucoma. Dr. Panarelli is certified by the American Board of Ophthalmology, and he is a member of the American Glaucoma Society as well as the American Academy of Ophthalmology. He received his Bachelor of Science in Finance from the Georgetown University McDonough School of Business in 2003 and his medical degree from the Georgetown University School of Medicine in 2007, where he was elected to the *Alpha Omega Alpha* Honor Medical Society during his junior year. He completed a residency in ophthalmology at the New York Eye and Ear Infirmary, where he served as chief resident during his final year of training. He was awarded the William and Judith Turner Award for excellence in ophthalmologic training. Following a year of fellowship training in glaucoma at the Bascom Palmer Eye Institute at the University of Miami Leonard M. Miller School of Medicine, he joined the faculty at Bascom Palmer for an additional year prior to returning to New York Eye and Ear Infirmary as a member of the full-time faculty. For 5 years there, he was active in resident education, serving as the associate residency program director as well as glaucoma fellowship director. Dr. Panarelli recently transitioned to New York University, where he serves as the chief in the Division of Glaucoma Services and director of the Glaucoma Fellowship. Dr. Panarelli is the recipient of several awards, including the Mentoring for Advancement of Physician-Scientist Award from the American Glaucoma Society, and he was selected as a *Castle Connolly Top Doctor* from 2017 to 2020. He has published extensively in his field and is a principal investigator for numerous studies pertaining to the surgical management of glaucoma.

ABOUT THE ASSOCIATE EDITORS

Davinder S. Grover, MD, MPH is an attending surgeon and clinician at Glaucoma Associates of Texas based in Dallas. His interests include innovative glaucoma surgeries, complex glaucoma, cataract and anterior segment surgeries, as well as clinical research outcomes in medical and surgical glaucoma. He has helped develop several innovative surgical techniques and has designed several novel surgical instruments. Dr. Grover also serves on the Board of Directors for the Cure Glaucoma Foundation, a charitable organization with a mission to improve access to quality care, fund transformational research, and disseminate knowledge through global outreach efforts.

He is the director of research at Glaucoma Associates of Texas. He has authored more than 40 peer-reviewed articles and more than 10 book chapters and has lectured around the world on glaucoma and innovative glaucoma surgeries.

Dr. Grover received his medical degree from The Johns Hopkins University School of Medicine in Baltimore, Maryland. He attended residency at the Wilmer Eye Institute at The Johns Hopkins Hospital and completed his glaucoma fellowship at the Bascom Palmer Eye Institute at the University of Miami Leonard M. Miller School of Medicine. Additionally, Dr. Grover also received a Master of Public Health degree at the Harvard T.H. Chan School of Public Health.

Arsham Sheybani, MD completed his medical degree with honors (AOA) at Washington University School of Medicine in St. Louis, Missouri. He then completed his residency in ophthalmology at Washington University in St. Louis and was selected to remain on faculty as chief resident. During that year, Dr. Sheybani was responsible for ophthalmologic trauma and emergencies as well as all adult inpatient ophthalmology consultations at Barnes-Jewish Hospital. He was the primary surgical teacher for the beginning residents and implemented a didactic system that is still used at Washington University. He then completed a fellowship with Iqbal "Ike" K. Ahmed in glaucoma and advanced anterior segment surgery in Toronto, Canada. He subsequently returned to Washington University School of Medicine as faculty in the Department of Ophthalmology and Visual Sciences, where he serves as residency program director. He has presented research internationally and is currently involved in device design aiming to make glaucoma surgery safer, among many other endeavors. He is an avid surgical teacher, winning the resident-selected faculty teaching award early in his career. He has also helped create one of the highest volume surgical glaucoma fellowships in the country, serving as the fellowship director.

CONTRIBUTING AUTHORS

Iqbal "Ike" K. Ahmed, MD (Chapters 9 and 17)
Assistant Professor, University of Toronto
Surgery Fellowship, University of Toronto
Fellowship Director, Glaucoma and Anterior Segment
Toronto, Ontario, Canada
Director of Research, Kensington Eye Institute
Head of Ophthalmology, Trillium Health Partners
Head of Innovation, Prism Eye Institute
Co-Medical Director, TLC Oakville
Ontario, Canada
Clinical Professor
University of Utah
Salt Lake City, Utah

Ahmad A. Aref, MD, MBA (Chapter 6)
Associate Professor of Ophthalmology and
Vice Chair for Clinical Affairs
Illinois Eye and Ear Infirmary
University of Illinois at Chicago College of Medicine
Chicago, Illinois

Lauren S. Blieden, MD (Chapter 15)
Associate Professor
Ophthalmology Department
Cullen Eye Institute
Baylor College of Medcine
Houston, Texas

Eileen C. Bowden, MD (Chapter 17)
Assistant Professor
Mitchel and Shannon Wong Eye Institute
University of Texas at Austin Dell Medical School
Austin, Texas

Donald L. Budenz, MD, MPH (Chapter 6)
Kittner Family Distinguished Professor and Chairman
Department of Ophthalmology
University of North Carolina
Chapel Hill, North Carolina

Teresa C. Chen, MD (Chapter 4)
Associate Professor of Ophthalmology
Department of Ophthalmology
Glaucoma Service
Massachusetts Eye and Ear
Harvard Medical School
Boston, Massachusetts

Panos G. Christakis, MD (Chapter 17)
Assistant Professor
Department of Ophthalmology & Vision Sciences
University of Toronto
Toronto, Ontario, Canada

Sara J. Coulon, MD (Chapters 3 and 8)
Resident Physician
Department of Ophthalmology
New York University
New York, New York

Sonal Dangda, MS (Ophthal) (Chapter 14)
Fellow
Pediatric Ophthalmology
Children's Mercy Hospital
Kansas City, Missouri

Anna T. Do, MD (Chapter 9)
Glaucoma and Cataract Surgeon
Eye Care of San Diego
San Diego, California

Murray Fingeret, OD (Chapter 8)
Clinical Professor
Clinical Science Department
State University of New York College of Optometry
New York, New York

Steven J. Gedde, MD (Chapters 14 and 17)
Professor of Ophthalmology and John G. Clarkson Chair
Vice Chairman of Education and Residency Program Director
Bascom Palmer Eye Institute
Miami, Florida

Jeffrey L. Goldberg, MD, PhD (Chapter 1)
Professor and Chair
Department of Ophthalmology
Byers Eye Institute at Stanford University
Palo Alto, California

J. Minjy Kang, MD (Chapter 7)
Assistant Professor
Ophthalmology Department
Northwestern University
Chicago, Illinois

Janice Kim, MD (Chapter 4)
Department of Ophthalmology
Edward S. Harkness Eye Institute
Columbia University Medical Center
New York, New York

Natasha Nayak Kolomeyer, MD (Chapter 13)
Assistant Professor of Glaucoma
Wills Eye Hospital
Thomas Jefferson University
Philadelphia, Pennsylvania

Rachel Lee, MD, MPH (Chapter 16)
Assistant Professor of Ophthalmology
Ophthalmology Department
New York Eye and Ear Infirmary of Mount Sinai
New York, New York

Wen-Shin Lee, MD (Chapter 1)
Clinical Assistant Professor
Ophthalmology Department
Byers Eye Institute at Stanford University
Palo Alto, California

Jonathan B. Lin, MD, PhD (Chapter 10)
Department of Ophthalmology
Massachusetts Eye and Ear
Harvard Medical School
Boston, Massachusetts

John T. Lind, MD, MS (Chapter 3)
Associate Professor of Ophthalmology
Director of Adult Clinical Ophthalmology
Associate Director of Medical Student Education
Department of Ophthalmology
Indiana University School of Medicine
Indianapolis, Indiana

Jonathan S. Myers, MD (Chapter 13)
Director
Glaucoma Service
Wills Eye Hospital
Thomas Jefferson University
Philadelphia, Pennsylvania

Lilian Nguyen, MD (Chapter 3)
Clinical Assistant Professor
Residency Associate Program Director
Medical Student Education
Department of Ophthalmology
University of Texas Health Science Center at San Antonio
San Antonio, Texas

Ravneet S. Rai, MD (Chapter 5)
Department of Ophthalmology
New York University Langone Health
New York, New York

Kitiya Ratanawongphaibul, MD (Chapter 4)
Faculty of Medicine
Glaucoma Research Unit
Chulalongkorn University
King Chulalongkorn Memorial Hospital
Thai Red Cross Society
Bangkok, Thailand

Joel S. Schuman, MD (Chapter 5)
Department of Ophthalmology
New York University Langone Health
New York, New York

R. Allan Sharpe, MD (Chapter 15)
Doctor of Glaucoma
Carolina Eye Associates
Southern Pines, North Carolina

Paul A. Sidoti, MD (Chapter 7)
Professor
Department of Ophthalmology
Icahn School of Medicine at Mount Sinai
New York Eye and Ear Infirmary of Mount Sinai
New York, New York

Kuldev Singh, MD, MPH (Chapter 16)
Professor of Ophthalmology
Director of Glaucoma Service
Ophthalmology Department
Byers Eye Institute at Stanford School of Medicine
Palo Alto, California

Kateki Vinod, MD (Chapter 2)
Assistant Professor
Department of Ophthalmology
Icahn School of Medicine at Mount Sinai
New York Eye and Ear Infirmary of Mount Sinai
New York, New York

Jing Wang, MD (Chapter 11)
Clinical Professor
Laval University
Quebec City, Quebec, Canada

Ruth D. Williams, MD (Chapter 17)
Glaucoma Consultant
Wheaton Eye Clinic
Wheaton, Illinois

Gadi Wollstein, MD (Chapter 5)
Department of Ophthalmology
New York University Langone Health
New York, New York

Eunmee Yook, MD (Chapter 12)
Glaucoma Specialist
Berkeley Eye Center
Houston, Texas

INTRODUCTION

The field of glaucoma continues to expand at a rapid pace. For the first time in more than a decade, we have several new US Food and Drug Administration–approved medications. A number of new surgical procedures have been developed and optimized to treat this challenging disease. Microinvasive glaucoma surgeries are best suited for patients with mild to moderate disease, whereas patients with advanced disease may be better served by our traditional glaucoma procedures. Multiple randomized prospective trials evaluating these procedures have been completed in recent years. These trials (as well as other recent landmark trials) provide the highest level of evidence, and specialists should be familiar with their results and understand how they can help guide their clinical practice. *The Pocket Guide to Glaucoma* is a concise, up-to-date resource for trainees as well as those who are just starting their career in ophthalmology. It is also well-suited for ophthalmologists who treat patients with glaucoma in their daily practice.

1

Glaucoma
Classification and Appropriate Terminology

Wen-Shin Lee, MD and Jeffrey L. Goldberg, MD, PhD

INTRODUCTION

Glaucoma is not a single disease entity, but rather a family of diseases with a shared endpoint: progressive degeneration and loss of the retinal ganglion cells and their axons with subsequent thinning of the optic nerve's neuroretinal rim.[1-3] This neuroretinal rim thinning results in a characteristic cupped appearance of the optic nerve in the glaucomatous eye. Because glaucoma encompasses a diverse set of diseases, organizing these diseases into a logical framework with consistent terminology is important to understanding glaucoma as a whole.

Elevated intraocular pressure (IOP) is the most important risk factor for the development and progression of optic nerve injury in glaucoma.[4-7] IOP is determined by the balance between aqueous humor production by the ciliary processes and aqueous humor outflow.[1,8] Elevated IOP in glaucoma generally occurs due to a decrease in aqueous outflow facility. Aqueous outflow occurs through 2 pathways.[9] The so-called *conventional* pathway accounts for the majority of aqueous outflow in the average eye.

Panarelli JF, ed.
The Pocket Guide to Glaucoma (pp 1-13).
© 2022 Taylor & Francis Group.

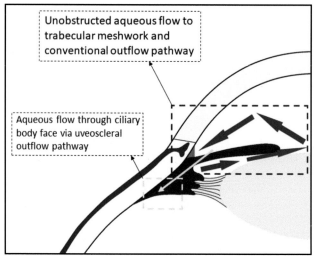

Unobstructed aqueous flow to trabecular meshwork and conventional outflow pathway

Aqueous flow through ciliary body face via uveoscleral outflow pathway

Figure 1-1. Open-angle configuration allowing free aqueous flow (blue arrows) to the iridocorneal angle. Also shown is the uveoscleral outflow pathway, which entails flow of aqueous across the ciliary body face and into the suprachoroidal space (yellow arrow).

In this pathway, the aqueous flows to the iridocorneal angle of the anterior chamber where it drains through the trabecular meshwork (TM), into Schlemm's canal, and eventually into the episcleral venous plexus (Figure 1-1). It is pressure-dependent. The second pathway, termed the *uveoscleral* pathway, encompasses flow of aqueous across the ciliary body face and into the suprachoroidal space, where it is eventually drained through the choroidal venous system (see Figure 1-1). This is pressure-independent outflow and may be responsible for 50% or more of aqueous outflow in younger, healthy eyes.

Glaucoma is broadly characterized based on the anatomy of the iridocorneal angle, which determines access to the conventional and, to some degree, the uveoscleral outflow pathways. Open-angle glaucoma (OAG) describes glaucoma in the setting of an iridocorneal angle in which there is no frank tissue obstruction of the pathway for aqueous to reach the TM (see Figure 1-1).

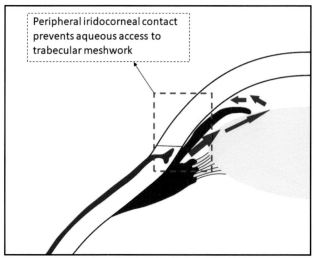

Peripheral iridocorneal contact prevents aqueous access to trabecular meshwork

Figure 1-2. Closed-angle configuration in which peripheral iridocorneal contact prevents aqueous flow (blue arrows) from reaching the TM and conventional outflow pathway.

In this setting, elevated IOP occurs due to decreased aqueous outflow facility despite free access to the TM.[1,8] Angle-closure glaucoma describes glaucoma in the setting of a mechanically obstructed iridocorneal angle, where contact between the peripheral iris and angle structures prevents aqueous from accessing the TM, thus resulting in elevated IOP[1,8] (Figure 1-2).

OPEN-ANGLE GLAUCOMA

Primary Open-Angle Glaucoma

Primary OAG (POAG) is defined by progressive neuroretinal rim thinning, optic nerve head cupping, and development of corresponding visual field defects in the setting of elevated IOP, but without identifiable cause of obstruction of the TM or distal outflow pathways.[1,8,9] The threshold for elevated IOP is typically set

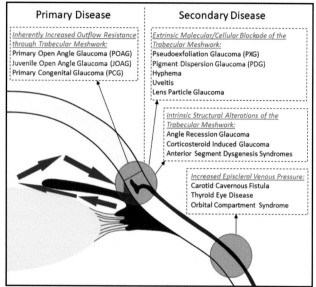

Primary Disease

Inherently Increased Outflow Resistance through Trabecular Meshwork:
Primary Open Angle Glaucoma (POAG)
Juvenile Open Angle Glaucoma (JOAG)
Primary Congenital Glaucoma (PCG)

Secondary Disease

Extrinsic Molecular/Cellular Blockade of the Trabecular Meshwork:
Pseudoexfoliation Glaucoma (PXG)
Pigment Dispersion Glaucoma (PDG)
Hyphema
Uveitis
Lens Particle Glaucoma

Intrinsic Structural Alterations of the Trabecular Meshwork:
Angle Recession Glaucoma
Corticosteroid Induced Glaucoma
Anterior Segment Dysgenesis Syndromes

Increased Episcleral Venous Pressure:
Carotid Cavernous Fistula
Thyroid Eye Disease
Orbital Compartment Syndrome

Figure 1-3. OAGs share a common endpoint of increased resistance to aqueous outflow with no frank tissue obstructing access to the iridocorneal angle and conventional outflow pathway. This increased outflow resistance can occur in the setting of no identifiable cause of outflow obstruction (primary disease), or an identifiable secondary cause of outflow obstruction (secondary disease), although primary disease likely also has molecular or cellular blockade yet to be identified.

at 21 mm Hg, which is 2 standard deviations above the Western population mean of 15.5 mm Hg.[10] The underlying cause for elevated IOP in POAG is theorized to be an age-related, degenerative change in the juxtacanalicular TM cells and extracellular matrix that results in increased outflow resistance[1,8,9] (Figure 1-3).

Normal-Tension Glaucoma

Normal-tension glaucoma (NTG; sometimes referred to as low tension glaucoma, given the nonspecific nature of the word "normal") is glaucoma that occurs at a statistically normal IOP (ie, <

21 mm Hg).[11] As with POAG, in NTG there is unobstructed access to the iridocorneal angle and no identifiable cause of obstruction of the conventional outflow pathway. The retinal ganglion cells and optic nerves of patients with NTG appear to be particularly susceptible to glaucomatous neurodegeneration. There is uncertainty regarding the threshold for "normal" IOP, given both the non-Gaussian distribution of IOP in population studies and the significant variation in IOP distribution that exists between demographic groups.[12-17] As such, NTG and POAG can be considered to exist along a spectrum with a common underlying pathophysiology, distinguished in most cases by the arbitrary distinction made based on IOP at presentation. In some cases, it is useful to remain aware of NTG as a separate entity; however, several distinct features of NTG suggest a greater contribution from non–IOP-related mechanisms, including associations with vasospastic disease and systemic hypotension, as well as increased rates of disc hemorrhages and early visual field defects closer to fixation.[18-21]

Secondary Open-Angle Glaucoma

Secondary OAGs occur in the absence of tissue obstructing access to the iridocorneal angle but with an identifiable secondary cause of increased outflow resistance through the TM or downstream collector channels that result in elevated IOP.[1,8] This group of diseases encompasses a variety of pathophysiologic mechanisms that converge on a common final endpoint of increased outflow resistance through the conventional outflow pathway (see Figure 1-3). Steroid-induced glaucoma is associated with IOP elevation in response to local or systemic steroids and is thought to be associated with a molecular buildup of extracellular matrix molecules in the TM.[22] When IOP rises further in a known POAG patient with topical or systemic steroid use, it is referred to as *steroid-response*. Entities such as pseudoexfoliation syndrome or pigment dispersion syndrome result in protein debris or pigment granules respectively in the anterior chamber, which can obstruct or impair the conventional outflow pathway as they are filtered upon exiting the eye.[23,24] Similarly, lens particle

glaucoma, phacolytic glaucoma, and phacoanaphylactic glaucoma block outflow with lens particles or reactive macrophages
or other immune cells, respectively.[9] A syndrome of recurrent,
nonscarring intraocular inflammation, called *iridocyclitic crisis*,
or *Posner-Schlossman syndrome*, presumably also overwhelms the
TM outflow pathway with immune cells and debris.[25]

Traumatic damage to the structures of the iridocorneal angle,
as occurs in angle recession, can result in an abnormal outflow
resistance due to post-traumatic damage to the structure of the
outflow pathway.[26] Orbital syndromes (thyroid eye disease) or
intracranial processes (carotid-cavernous fistula) can result in
increased episcleral venous pressure, which leads to increased
resistance to aqueous flow out of the eye.[27]

ANGLE-CLOSURE GLAUCOMA

Primary Angle-Closure Disease

In angle-closure glaucomas, there is an iris-based mechanical
apposition and obstruction of the iridocorneal angle. Primary
angle-closure (PAC) disease encompasses a spectrum of anatomy
in which the peripheral iris and TM come together due to the
inherent anatomy of an individual eye[28] (Figure 1-4). Anatomic
features that underlie PAC include shorter axial length of the eye,
increased iris thickness, anterior rotation of the ciliary body (plateau iris configuration), and increased lens thickness/increased
anterior lens vault (phacomorphic glaucoma).[29-32] These features
can lead to appositional closure of the iridocorneal angle and
are further divided into pupillary block and nonpupillary block
mechanisms. This appositional angle closure can be acute, with
a sudden elevation in IOP that does not resolve spontaneously,
or subacute, with intermittent elevations in IOP that spontaneously resolve. Chronic angle closure, on the other hand, describes
the gradual development of peripheral anterior synechiae (PAS)
between peripheral iris and TM that have been in chronic apposition and/or subjected to inflammation and scarring, which can
ultimately result in irreversible closure of the iridocorneal angle.

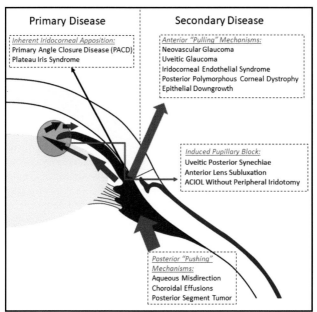

Figure 1-4. The angle-closure glaucomas share a common endpoint of decreased aqueous outflow facility resulting from the inability of aqueous flow to reach the TM due to peripheral iridocorneal contact. This peripheral iridocorneal contact, and eventual PAS formation, can be due to the inherent anatomical features of the eye (primary disease), or a variety of disease mechanisms that pull the peripheral iris anteriorly, push the peripheral iris anteriorly, or induce pupillary block (secondary disease).

The contemporary classification of PAC disease divides this spectrum of anatomy into 3 categories: PAC suspect, PAC, and PAC glaucoma.[28] PAC suspect is defined as an eye with > 180 degrees of apposition between the peripheral iris and TM on gonioscopy, but no elevation in IOP, no PAS, and no evidence of glaucomatous optic neuropathy. PAC is defined as an eye that meets the criteria for PAC suspect, but additionally has an elevated IOP or PAS. PAC glaucoma is defined as an eye that meets the criteria for PAC, but additionally demonstrates evidence of glaucomatous optic neuropathy.

Secondary Angle-Closure Glaucoma

Apposition between the peripheral iris and TM can also be observed secondary to an identifiable pathophysiologic mechanism rather than the primary anatomic features of an eye[33] (see Figure 1-4). Such secondary angle-closure glaucoma (SACG) can be broadly categorized into disease processes anterior to the iris that pull the peripheral iris forward, or disease processes posterior to the iris that push the peripheral iris forward. Additionally, SACG can result from pathology at the pupillary margin of the iris itself inducing pupillary block, including posterior synechiae between the iris and anterior lens capsule in the setting of uveitis, anterior subluxation of the crystalline lens, and anterior chamber intraocular lens placement without a peripheral iridotomy.

SACG due to pathology anterior to the iris includes neovascular glaucoma, uveitic glaucoma, iridocorneal endothelial syndrome, posterior polymorphous corneal dystrophy, and epithelial downgrowth.[9,33-36] This set of diseases can produce anterior synechiae between the peripheral iris and TM independent of preceding anatomic apposition between these structures. SACG due to pathology posterior to the iris, on the other hand, is due to anatomic apposition between the peripheral iris and TM from an identifiable mechanism pushing the iris anteriorly toward the iridocorneal angle. This includes posterior segment tumors, malignant glaucoma, and large choroidal effusions.[9,33,37,38]

PEDIATRIC GLAUCOMA

Glaucoma in children follows similar pathophysiologic principles to glaucoma in adults, with decreased aqueous humor outflow facility resulting in elevated IOP and subsequent retinal ganglion cell injury. Pediatric glaucoma is classified by both age of onset and the underlying mechanism for decreased aqueous outflow.[39-41]

Glaucoma that occurs before the age of 4 years is termed *congenital* glaucoma. Glaucoma that occurs between the ages of 4 to 35 years is termed *juvenile* glaucoma. Congenital glaucoma can further be divided into neonatal, infantile, and late onset categories based on the age of onset (< 1 month, < 2 years, and 2 to 4 years of age, respectively).[39,41]

Primary Congenital Glaucoma

Primary congenital glaucoma (PCG) is generally thought to be due to a primary and isolated developmental anomaly of the iridocorneal angle structures.[39,41] This anomalous angle anatomy is described by the term *trabeculodysgenesis*, and gonioscopically can be characterized by indistinct angle structures with direct insertion of the iris onto the TM.[42,43] Children with PCG do not have contributory systemic syndromes, broader ocular dysgenesis syndromes, or prior ocular surgery.

Juvenile Open-Angle Glaucoma

Juvenile OAG (JOAG) is similar to POAG but presenting in the pediatric population, with normal-appearing angle structures on gonioscopy, and the absence of contributory systemic syndromes or broader ocular dysgenesis syndromes.[41,44] It is postulated that JOAG, like POAG, occurs due to an inherent abnormality in resistance to aqueous outflow through the TM despite a normal macroscopic appearance. JOAG can be distinguished from a late diagnosis of PCG by the absence of IOP-induced changes in the eye, such as buphthalmos, megalocornea, and Haab striae, which typically do not occur after 4 years of age.[44]

Secondary Childhood Glaucomas

As with adults, glaucoma in children that results from decreased aqueous outflow due to a mechanism other than an isolated and primary anomaly of the conventional outflow pathway is deemed secondary glaucoma. This group of diseases can be broadly classified into glaucoma due to a broader ocular dysgenesis syndrome, glaucoma due to acquired ocular disease, glaucoma secondary to a systemic disorder, and glaucoma due to prior cataract surgery.[41]

Broader ocular dysgenesis syndromes include entities such as aniridia, Axenfeld-Rieger syndrome, and Peters anomaly.[45-47] These syndromes manifest with anomalies of the lens, iris, and cornea in addition to the iridocorneal angle and TM. Acquired ocular diseases that can secondarily result in elevated IOP include entities such as retinopathy of prematurity and uveitis.[48,49] Systemic disorders that include ocular anomalies that can result in elevated IOP include entities such as Sturge-Weber syndrome and Weill-Marchesani syndrome.[50,51] Finally, extraction of a pediatric cataract has shown a strong association with subsequent IOP elevation, which is often described as aphakic or pseudophakic glaucoma.[52]

CONCLUSION

Taken together, glaucoma classification is still imperfect, particularly when it comes to molecular or genetic definition and understanding for most cases. Nevertheless, because there are fine points of medical and surgical treatment that differ in efficacy between these glaucomas, and to facilitate ongoing research into the pathophysiology and treatment of disease, careful clinical examination and differentiation into these classifications remains an important mainstay of clinical practice.

REFERENCES

1.   Quigley HA. Glaucoma. *Lancet.* 2011;377(9774):1367-1377.
2.   Quigley HA, Dunkelberger GR, Green WR. Retinal ganglion cell atrophy correlated with automated perimetry in human eyes with glaucoma. *Am J Ophthalmol.* 1989;107(5):453-464.
3.   Foster PJ, Buhrmann R, Quigley HA, Johnson GJ. The definition and classification of glaucoma in prevalence surveys. *Br J Ophthalmol.* 2002;86(2):238-242.

4.   Gordon MO, Beiser JA, Brandt JD, et al. The Ocular Hypertension Treatment Study: baseline factors that predict the onset of primary open-angle glaucoma. *Arch Ophthalmol.* 2002;120(6):714-720.

5.   Coleman AL, Miglior S. Risk factors for glaucoma onset and progression. *Surv Ophthalmol.* 2008;53(Suppl 1):S3-S10.

6.   Leske MC, Heijl A, Hussein M, et al. Factors for glaucoma progression and the effect of treatment: the early manifest glaucoma trial. *Arch Ophthalmol.* 2003;121(1):48-56.

7.   Leske MC, Heijl A, Hyman L, et al. Predictors of long-term progression in the early manifest glaucoma trial. *Ophthalmology.* 2007;114(11):1965-1972.

8.   Jonas JB, Aung T, Bourne RR, et al. Glaucoma. *Lancet.* 2017;390(10108):2183-2193.

9.   American Academy of Ophthalmology. *Basic and Clinical Science Course. Glaucoma, Section 10.* Author; 2014:16-19.

10. Colton T, Ederer F. The distribution of intraocular pressures in the general population. *Surv Ophthalmol.* 1980;25(3):123-129.

11. Killer HE, Pircher A. Normal tension glaucoma: review of current understanding and mechanisms of the pathogenesis. *Eye (Lond).* 2018;32(5):924-930.

12. Dielemans I, Vingerling JR, Wolfs RC, et al. The prevalence of primary open-angle glaucoma in a population-based study in the Netherlands. The Rotterdam Study. *Ophthalmology.* 1994;101(11):1851-1855.

13. Bonomi L, Marchini G, Marraffa M, et al. Prevalence of glaucoma and intraocular pressure distribution in a defined population. The Egna-Neumarkt Study. *Ophthalmology.* 1998;105(2):209-215.

14. Iwase A, Suzuki Y, Araie M, et al. The prevalence of primary open-angle glaucoma in Japanese: the Tajimi Study. *Ophthalmology.* 2004;111(9):1641-1648.

15. He M, Foster PJ, Ge J, et al. Prevalence and clinical characteristics of glaucoma in adult Chinese: a population-based study in Liwan District, Guangzhou. *Invest Ophthalmol Vis Sci.* 2006;47(7):2782-2788.

16. Kim CS, Seong GJ, Lee NH, et al. Prevalence of primary open-angle glaucoma in central South Korea: the Namil study. *Ophthalmology.* 2011;118(6):1024-1030.

17. Rotchford AP, Johnson GJ. Glaucoma in Zulus: a population-based cross-sectional survey in a rural district in South Africa. *Arch Ophthalmol.* 2002;120(4):471-478.

18. Flammer J. The vascular concept of glaucoma. *Surv Ophthalmol.* 1994;38(Suppl):S3-S6.

19. Meyer JH, Brandi-Dohrn J, Funk J. Twenty four hour blood pressure monitoring in normal tension glaucoma. *Br J Ophthalmol.* 1996;80(10):864-867.

20. Caprioli J, Sears M, Spaeth GL. Comparison of visual field defects in normal-tension glaucoma and high-tension glaucoma. *Am J Ophthalmol.* 1986;102(3):402-404.

21. Thonginnetra O, Greenstein VC, Chu D, et al. Normal versus high tension glaucoma: a comparison of functional and structural defects. *J Glaucoma.* 2010;19(3):151-157.

22. Razeghinejad MR, Katz LJ. Steroid-induced iatrogenic glaucoma. *Ophthalmic Res.* 2012;47(2):66-80.

23. Plateroti P, Plateroti AM, Abdolrahimzadeh S, Scuderi G. Pseudoexfoliation syndrome and pseudoexfoliation glaucoma: a review of the literature with updates on surgical management. *J Ophthalmol.* 2015;2015:370371.

24. Yang JW, Sakiyalak D, Krupin T. Pigmentary glaucoma. *J Glaucoma.* 2001;10(5 Suppl 1):S30-S32. Review.

25. Megaw R, Agarwal PK. Posner-Schlossman syndrome. *Surv Ophthalmol.* 2017;62(3):277-285.

26. Bai HQ, Yao L, Wang DB, Jin R, Wang YX. Causes and treatments of traumatic secondary glaucoma. *Eur J Ophthalmol.* 2009;19(2):201-206.

27. Greenfield DS. Glaucoma associated with elevated episcleral venous pressure. *J Glaucoma.* 2000;9(2):190-194.

28. Razeghinejad MR, Myers JS. Contemporary approach to the diagnosis and management of primary angle-closure disease. *Surv Ophthalmol.* 2018;63(6):754-768.

29. Lowe RF. Aetiology of the anatomical basis for primary angle-closure glaucoma. Biometrical comparisons between normal eyes and eyes with primary angle-closure glaucoma. *Br J Ophthalmol.* 1970;54(3):161-169.

30. Lee RY, Kasuga T, Cui QN, et al. Association between baseline iris thickness and prophylactic laser peripheral iridotomy outcomes in primary angle-closure suspects. *Ophthalmology.* 2014;121(6):1194-1202.

31. Lan YW, Hsieh JW, Hung PT. Ocular biometry in acute and chronic angle-closure glaucoma. *Ophthalmologica.* 2007;221(6):388-394.

32. Tan GS, He M, Zhao W, et al. Determinants of lens vault and association with narrow angles in patients from Singapore. *Am J Ophthalmol.* 2012;154(1):39-46.

33. Parivadhini A, Lingam V. Management of secondary angle closure glaucoma. *J Curr Glaucoma Pract.* 2014;8(1):25-32.

34. Havens SJ, Gulati V. Neovascular glaucoma. *Dev Ophthalmol.* 2016;55:196-204.

35. Siddique SS, Suelves AM, Baheti U, Foster CS. Glaucoma and uveitis. *Surv Ophthalmol.* 2013;58(1):1-10.

36. Silva L, Najafi A, Suwan Y, Teekhasaenee C, Ritch R. The iridocorneal endothelial syndrome. *Surv Ophthalmol.* 2018;63(5):665-676.

37. Kaplowitz K, Yung E, Flynn R, Tsai JC. Current concepts in the treatment of vitreous block, also known as aqueous misdirection. *Surv Ophthalmol.* 2015;60(3):229-241.

38. Murphy RM, Bakir B, O'Brien C, Wiggs JL, Pasquale LR. Drug-induced bilateral secondary angle-closure glaucoma: a literature synthesis. *J Glaucoma.* 2016;25(2):e99-e105.

39. Yu Chan JY, Choy BN, Ng AL, Shum JW. Review on the management of primary congenital glaucoma. *J Curr Glaucoma Pract.* 2015;9(3):92-99.

40. Ko F, Papadopoulos M, Khaw PT. Primary congenital glaucoma. *Prog Brain Res.* 2015;221:177-189.

41. Thau A, Lloyd M, Freedman S, et al. New classification system for pediatric glaucoma: implications for clinical care and a research registry. *Curr Opin Ophthalmol.* 2018;29(5):385-394.

42. Anderson DR. The development of the trabecular meshwork and its abnormality in primary infantile glaucoma. *Trans Am Ophthalmol Soc.* 1981;79:458-485.

43. Maul E, Strozzi L, Muñoz C, Reyes C. The outflow pathway in congenital glaucoma. *Am J Ophthalmol.* 1980;89(5):667-673.

44. Turalba AV, Chen TC. Clinical and genetic characteristics of primary juvenile-onset open-angle glaucoma (JOAG). *Semin Ophthalmol.* 2008;23(1):19-25.

45. Balekudaru S, Sankaranarayanan N, Agarkar S. Prevalence, incidence, and risk factors for the development of glaucoma in patients with aniridia. *J Pediatr Ophthalmol Strabismus.* 2017;54(4):250-255.

46. Chang TC, Summers CG, Schimmenti LA, Grajewski AL. Axenfeld-Rieger syndrome: new perspectives. *Br J Ophthalmol.* 2012;96(3):318-322.

47. Bhandari R, Ferri S, Whittaker B, Liu M, Lazzaro DR. Peters anomaly: review of the literature. *Cornea.* 2011;30(8):939-944.

48. Bremer DL, Rogers DL, Good WV, et al. Glaucoma in the Early Treatment for Retinopathy of Prematurity (ETROP) study. *J AAPOS.* 2012;16(5):449-452.

49. Kaur S, Kaushik S, Singh Pandav S. Pediatric uveitic glaucoma. *J Curr Glaucoma Pract.* 2013;7(3):115-117.

50. Mantelli F, Bruscolini A, La Cava M, Abdolrahimzadeh S, Lambiase A. Ocular manifestations of Sturge-Weber syndrome: pathogenesis, diagnosis, and management. *Clin Ophthalmol.* 2016;10:871-878.

51. Senthil S, Rao HL, Hoang NT, et al. Glaucoma in microspherophakia: presenting features and treatment outcomes. *J Glaucoma.* 2014;23(4):262-267.

52. Trivedi RH, Wilson ME Jr, Golub RL. Incidence and risk factors for glaucoma after pediatric cataract surgery with and without intraocular lens implantation. *J AAPOS.* 2006;10(2):117-123.

2

What Is Glaucoma and Who Is At Risk for It?

Kateki Vinod, MD

INTRODUCTION

Glaucoma encompasses a group of diseases characterized by progressive optic neuropathy with the potential for irreversible blindness if untreated. Recognizable changes in optic nerve structure and function as demonstrated by clinical examination and supplemental imaging (ie, optical coherence tomography retinal nerve fiber layer and perimetry) typify glaucoma. While an important risk factor, intraocular pressure (IOP) is only one of many contributors to the development of glaucoma. Glaucoma may be classified according to various features, including anatomical configuration (eg, open-angle vs closed-angle glaucoma) and etiology (eg, primary vs secondary glaucoma). Clinical manifestations vary greatly based on glaucoma subtype, with some arising insidiously and without symptoms and others acutely with exquisite pain, redness, and blurred vision. Glaucoma is a major public health burden and the second leading cause of blindness worldwide.[1] It is projected to affect 111.8 million people globally in the year 2040.[2]

Panarelli JF, ed.
The Pocket Guide to Glaucoma (pp 15-23).
© 2022 Taylor & Francis Group.

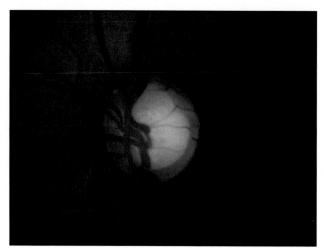

Figure 2-1A. Focal superior notch in the left optic nerve head of a patient with juvenile open-angle glaucoma.

ANATOMY AND PATHOPHYSIOLOGY

The normal optic nerve head is composed of approximately 1.2 to 1.5 million axons (nerve fibers) arising from retinal ganglion cells (RGCs), which traverse the fenestrated lamina cribrosa en route to the lateral geniculate body. Nerve fibers originating from the temporal peripheral retina (arcuate fibers) reach the optic nerve head via an arc-like route from above and below the median (horizontal) raphe, while those arising from the macula (papillomacular fibers) and nasal peripheral retina have a more direct course.

Despite their diverse histopathologic and clinical features, all glaucomas share the common endpoint of progressive optic neuropathy resulting from apoptosis of RGCs and their axonal loss. Glaucomatous optic nerve heads are characterized by the loss of optic nerve fibers from the neural rim, resulting in increased cup-to-disc ratio due either to focal (Figure 2-1) or diffuse atrophy

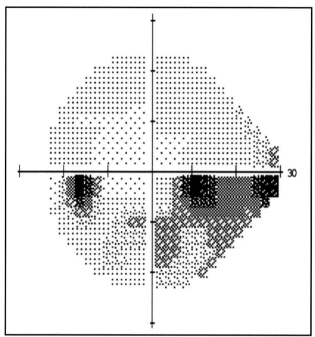

Figure 2-1B. Corresponding visual field of the left eye demonstrating an inferior nasal step.

(Figure 2-2). The superior and inferior poles of the optic nerve head appear to be most vulnerable to glaucomatous damage. The ISNT (inferior rim thickness > superior > nasal > temporal) rule is an oft-used principle for identifying normal vs abnormal optic nerve head cupping. Disruption of the normal progression of rim width thickness should alert the clinician to the presence of glaucoma. Localized (wedge) or diffuse loss of peripapillary nerve fiber bundles may be clinically visible adjacent to the site of neural rim thinning. Nonglaucomatous optic neuropathies classically demonstrate neural rim pallor, usually out of proportion to cupping, which helps to distinguish them from glaucomatous

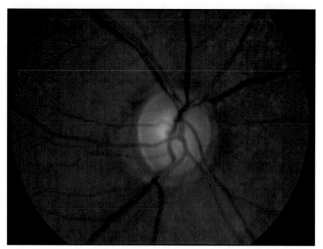

Figure 2-2. Diffuse optic atrophy with pronounced inferior greater than superior thinning of the neural rim in a patient with primary open-angle glaucoma.

optic neuropathy. Patients with advanced glaucoma exhibit complete loss of neural rim tissue with posterior bowing and greater prominence of the lamina cribrosa, which can occasionally be mistaken for pallor (Figure 2-3). Transient, linear (Drance) optic nerve hemorrhages (Figure 2-4) located in or near the neural rim serve as harbingers of subsequent retinal nerve fiber layer loss and visual field defects. Nasalization of blood vessels and the presence of choriocapillaris and retinal pigment epithelium peripapillary (beta-zone) atrophy are also seen in glaucoma. The loss of RGCs and their nerve fibers as they course toward particular locations on the optic nerve head usually correspond to predictable patterns of visual field loss (see Chapter 6).

The pathophysiology of glaucoma is complex and not completely understood. The characteristic appearance of the glaucomatous optic nerve head suggests that the nerve itself, rather than the retina, is the primary site of damage in glaucoma.[3] An early "mechanical" theory suggested that elevated IOP caused direct compression of the optic nerve head, leading to cupping.

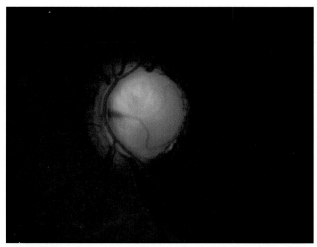

Figure 2-3. Advanced cupping in a patient with juvenile open-angle glaucoma. Note the near total loss of neural rim.

An opposing vascular theory proposed that abnormal perfusion and resultant ischemia were responsible for glaucomatous optic neuropathy. Vascular dysregulation may also contribute to compromised perfusion of the optic nerve head, either due to elevated IOP or IOP-independent alterations in systemic hemodynamics. Animal studies have demonstrated IOP-induced disruption to axoplasmic flow at the level of the lamina cribrosa,[4] but data are conflicting as to whether this phenomenon results from mechanical or vascular factors. Potential contributions of systemic blood pressure and intracranial pressure to glaucomatous damage have garnered attention in recent years and are under investigation.

RISK FACTORS

Risk factors for glaucoma vary according to subtype, though some, like IOP, are important in all glaucomas. IOP elevation results from increased resistance to aqueous outflow caused by

Figure 2-4A. Inferotemporal splinter hemorrhage in a patient with preperimetric open-angle glaucoma of the left eye.

anatomical angle closure or, in an open angle, ultrastructural changes within the trabecular meshwork and/or downstream pathways. After Eddy and Billings' 1988 report pronouncing the lack of evidence regarding the efficacy of glaucoma treatment,[5] several landmark clinical trials were conducted that demonstrated the benefit of IOP-lowering therapy on glaucomatous development and progression (see Chapter 17). IOP remains the only modifiable risk factor for glaucoma and its reduction is the only proven treatment method. However, IOP-independent factors, such as systemic hypotension and vascular dysregulation, also play a role in the pathogenesis of glaucoma, especially that of normal-tension glaucoma.

In general, glaucoma develops more frequently in people of older age. Primary open-angle glaucoma (POAG) has been shown to be more than 10 times more prevalent in patients aged 80 years or older compared with those aged 40 to 49 years.[6,7] Of note, however, POAG manifests much earlier in patients of African

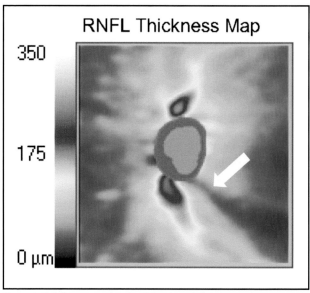

Figure 2-4B. Inferotemporal wedge defect (arrow) demonstrated on Cirrus optical coherence tomography retinal nerve fiber layer in the same patient as Figure 2-4A indicates a peripapillary nerve fiber bundle defect 1 year after the observed disc hemorrhage.

and Afro-Caribbean descent vs those of European descent, and warrants screening efforts in younger patients. A study of Haitian patients in South Florida found a prevalence of glaucoma suspect status (ie, IOP ≥ 24 mm Hg, vertical cup-to-disc ratio ≥ 0.7, and/or clinical evidence of glaucomatous optic nerve damage in at least 1 eye) of 20.9% in those aged 18 to 40 years.[8] Primary angle-closure glaucoma (PACG) is more common in older age, in part due to the forward displacement of a growing cataractous lens.

Ethnicity may increase the risk of developing certain subtypes of glaucoma. The Baltimore Eye Survey noted a 3- to 4-fold higher prevalence of POAG among Black patients as compared with White patients across nearly all age intervals.[7] Hiller and Kahn noted a 7-fold higher rate of blindness among non-White patients with glaucoma (of whom 97.5% were Black patients) than in White patients of all ages in the United States.[9] Hispanic patients aged 80 or older also demonstrate a much higher prevalence of POAG than White patients of the same age.[10] Meanwhile, the risk of PACG is highest among certain Inuit[11] and East Asian populations,[2] and Japanese patients show an increased prevalence of normal-tension glaucoma.[12]

Myopia and insulin resistance are among other risk factors for POAG that are under study. Additional anatomical features that predispose eyes to PACG include hyperopia, short axial length, and shallow anterior chamber, while physiologic features include thicker irides, greater iris volume retention after dilation, and choroidal expansion.[13] The genetic basis of different subtypes of glaucoma is not yet well elucidated, but a history of glaucoma in a first-degree relative appears to confer risk for both POAG and PACG.

Numerous secondary glaucomas exist for which anatomic, physiologic, and environmental risk factors are more specific. For example, proliferative diabetic retinopathy and retinal venous (and less commonly arterial) occlusions can lead to retinal ischemia, which in turn can incite neovascular glaucoma. Other secondary glaucomas include those related to the lens, uveitis, trauma, steroid use, and melanoma, as well as pigmentary and pseudoexfoliation glaucomas (see Chapter 1).

CONCLUSION

The glaucomas are a large group of complex diseases whose pathogenesis is multifactorial and whose risk factors are numerous. Early detection and treatment of clinically distinguishable changes in the structure of the optic nerve head may help prevent visual field loss and blindness. While one of many risk factors, IOP is the only contributor that can be modified and IOP lowering is therefore the goal of current glaucoma treatment. Further studies regarding the underlying genetic basis and molecular mechanisms of glaucoma may lead to the development of more targeted therapies in the future.

REFERENCES

1. Kingman S. Glaucoma is second leading cause of blindness globally. *Bull World Health Organ.* 2004;82:887-888.

2. Tham YC, Li X, Wong TY, et al. Global prevalence of glaucoma and projections of glaucoma burden through 2040: a systematic review and meta-analysis. *Ophthalmology.* 2014;121(11):2081-2090.

3. Hayreh SS. The blood supply of the optic nerve head and the evaluation of it—myth and reality. *Prog Retin Eye Res.* 2001;20(5):563-593.

4. Anderson DR, Hendrickson A. Effect of intraocular pressure on rapid axoplasmic transport in monkey optic nerve. *Invest Ophthalmol.* 1974;13(10):771-783.

5. Eddy DM, Billings J. The quality of medical evidence: implications for quality of care. *Health Aff (Millwood).* 1988;7(1):19-32.

6. Friedman DS, Wolfs RC, O'Colmain BJ, et al. Prevalence of open-angle glaucoma among adults in the United States. *Arch Ophthalmol.* 2004;122(4):532-538.

7. Tielsch JM, Sommer A, Katz J, et al. Racial variations in the prevalence of primary open-angle glaucoma. The Baltimore Eye Survey. *JAMA.* 1991;266(3):369-374.

8. Bokman CL, Pasquale LR, Parrish RK 2nd, et al. Glaucoma screening in the Haitian Afro-Caribbean population of South Florida. *PLoS One.* 2014;9(12):e115942.

9. Hiller R, Kahn HA. Blindness from glaucoma. *Am J Ophthalmol.* 1975;80(1):62-69.

10. Quigley HA, West SK, Rodriguez J, et al. The prevalence of glaucoma in a population-based study of Hispanic subjects: Proyecto VER. *Arch Ophthalmol.* 2001;119(12):1819-1826.

11. Congdon N, Wang F, Tielsch JM. Issues in the epidemiology and population-based screening of primary angle-closure glaucoma. *Surv Ophthalmol.* 1992;36(6):411-423.

12. Suzuki Y, Iwase A, Araie M, et al. Risk factors for open-angle glaucoma in a Japanese population: the Tajimi Study. *Ophthalmology.* 2006;113(9):1613-1617.

13. Quigley HA. Angle-closure glaucoma—simpler answers to complex mechanisms: LXVI Edward Jackson Memorial Lecture. *Am J Ophthalmol.* 2009;148(5):657-669.e1.

3

Measuring Intraocular Pressure

Lilian Nguyen, MD; John T. Lind, MD, MS;
and Sara J. Coulon, MD

INTRODUCTION

Glaucoma is a chronic and progressive optic neuropathy, with many contributing factors to its development. Intraocular pressure (IOP), however, remains the only important modifiable risk factor.

Numerous landmark studies have shown the importance of IOP control in glaucoma. The Ocular Hypertension Treatment Study found more than a 50% risk reduction in the conversion to glaucoma at 5 years when the IOP was reduced by 22.5%.[1] The Early Manifest Glaucoma Trial randomized patients with newly diagnosed disease to observation or medical/laser treatment; at 5 years, the risk of glaucomatous progression was 62% in the observation group and 45% in the treatment group.[2] The Collaborative Initial Glaucoma Treatment Study randomized patients with newly diagnosed disease of varying severity to either medical therapy or surgical intervention with a more aggressive IOP target and found that neither group showed visual field progression after 5 years of follow-up.[3]

Panarelli JF, ed.
The Pocket Guide to Glaucoma (pp 25-37).
© 2022 Taylor & Francis Group.

Evidence demonstrates that reduction of IOP can reduce the risk of developing glaucomatous changes and progression of the disease. For this reason, many devices with various methods of action have been developed to estimate IOP. Different methods of tonometry include applanation, dynamic contour, rebound, indentation, noncontact, Ocular Response Analyzer (ORA; Reichert Technologies), digital, and transpalpebral. This chapter will focus on the different devices available.

APPLANATION

Goldmann Applanation Tonometry

Goldmann applanation tonometry (GAT) is considered the gold standard for measuring IOP. Applanation estimating IOP is based on the Imbert-Fick principle, which states that the pressure inside an ideal, dry, thin-walled sphere equals the force necessary to flatten its surface divided by the area of the flattening. Goldmann modified the equation to account for the resistance of the cornea to applanation and the action of surface tension from the tear meniscus on the tonometer prism.

The GAT is slit lamp mounted. Topical anesthetic and fluorescein dye are instilled into the tear film. When viewed through the slit lamp with a cobalt blue filter, the tonometer bi-prism splits the image of the fluorescent tear meniscus into 2 semicircular rings. A dial on the side of the tonometer is adjusted to vary the force applied to the eye, causing a movement of the rings until the inner edges of the semicircles touch each other, estimating an IOP measured in mm Hg.

Disadvantages of the GAT method include high skill level to operate, need for topical anesthesia, inability to use on supine patients, difficulty with children or those unable to sit at slit lamp, and decreased accuracy with irregular or scarred corneas.

Of note, since Goldmann applanation tonometry is the standard-of-care IOP measurement device, most devices are compared to it when determining accuracy.

Perkins Tonometer

The Perkins tonometer (Haag-Streit Holding) is a type of portable applanation tonometer. It is a hand-held device that is useful in situations where a slit lamp exam is not feasible. There is high agreement between the Perkins tonometer and the GAT, with a mean difference of 1.0 mm Hg between the 2 tonometers. It can be used for patients in the supine position (useful in children during examinations under anesthesia).

Disadvantages of this method are similar to the GAT method: high skill level to operate, need for topical anesthetic, and decreased accuracy with irregular or scarred corneas.[4-6]

Tono-Pen Applanation Tonometer

The Tono-Pen (Reichert Technologies) is a portable, lightweight, electronic applanation tonometer. It contains a gauge that senses the force generated to indent the central cornea, similar to GAT methodology (Figure 3-1). The digital readout is an average of at least 4 IOP measurements with a coefficient of variation. The manufacturer recommends the coefficient of variation be less than 5% to be considered accurate.

Advantages of the Tono-Pen are its ease of use and transportability. Also, due to its small contact area as compared to the GAT, it is useful for IOP measurements in irregular corneas. However, studies have shown that the Tono-Pen overestimates and underestimates IOP compared to GAT without a consistent pattern. Thus, it is best used with caution and should be supplemented by a different method when possible.[7-9]

DYNAMIC CONTOUR TONOMETRY

The dynamic contour device is a digital, nonapplanation, slit lamp mounted, contact tonometer that may be more independent of corneal biomechanical properties and thickness than older tonometers. The dynamic contour tonometry (DCT) has

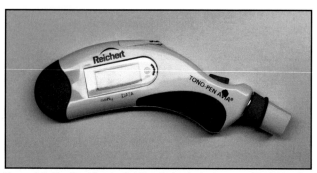

Figure 3-1. The Tono-Pen by Reichert Technologies is a portable device that measures the force required to indent the cornea.

a contoured tonometer tip surface that matches the same shape as the corneal curvature with a miniature pressure sensor in its center. The probe is placed on the precorneal tear film, and the integrated pressure sensor automatically begins to acquire data, measuring IOP 100 times per second.

The DCT provides a quality score of the IOP measurement ranging from 1 (optimum) to 5 (unacceptable). For clinical purposes, the manufacturer suggests quality scores of 1 or 2. Most studies suggest that DCT overestimates GAT by ~2 to 3 mm Hg, depending on central corneal thickness (CCT) and IOP. Research has suggested optimal use in certain clinical situations, such as keratoconus, corneal edema, and postpenetrating keratoplasty or refractive corneal surgery.[8,10-17]

REBOUND TONOMETRY

Rebound tonometry uses a dynamic electromechanical method for measuring IOP by bouncing a small plastic tipped metal probe against the cornea. The device consists of a solenoid propelling coil and a sensing coil positioned around a central shaft containing a lightweight magnetized probe. The application of a transient electrical current to the solenoid coil propels the probe to the cornea. As the probe impacts cornea, it decelerates and rebounds from the surface and back into the device, creating an induction current from which the IOP is calculated.

The iCare is a commercial rebound tonometer that is a hand-held device, and corneal anesthesia is not required. On activation of the measurement button, it automatically takes 6 readings of IOP and presents a digital readout of the mean IOP. This device is particularly useful when measuring IOP in young children. In many pediatric ophthalmology practices, this device has decreased the frequency of IOP checks under anesthesia, as many young patients tolerate this device well.

Research about the iCare's accuracy have been conflicting. Van der Jagt and Jansonius found that iCare overestimated GAT by 0.6 mm Hg, though the difference was not significant. Nakamura et al, however, demonstrated that iCare overestimated GAT by 1.40 ± 4.29 mm Hg, but that this was dependent on CCT. Overall, the general consensus among glaucoma professionals is that iCare is a reasonable option for IOP measurement, as it is in close agreement with GAT in clinical practice.[18-22]

INDENTATION TONOMETRY

Pneumotonometry

The pneumatic tonometer, or Pneumatonometer (Reichert Technologies), utilizes aspects of both applanation and indentation tonometry. It has a pressure-sensing device that consists of a gas-filled chamber covered with a silicone diaphragm (Figure 3-2). As the diaphragm touches the cornea, the gas vent decreases in size and the pressure in the chamber rises until the cornea and tip are flat, and this is used to calculate the IOP. Pneumotonometry tends to underestimate GAT at lower IOP and overestimate GAT when the IOP is high.[23]

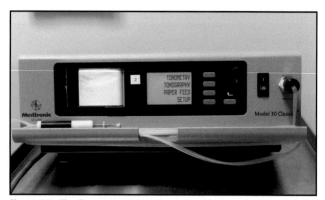

Figure 3-2. The Pneumatonometer uses a combination of applanation and indentation tonometry. It has a pressure-sensing device that consists of a gas-filled chamber covered with a silicone diaphragm to measure pressure. These readings correlate with GAT when pressures are in a normal range.

Schiotz Tonometer

The Schiotz tonometer requires corneal anesthesia and is used with patients in the supine position. A weighted plunger attached to a curved footplate that sits on the cornea is allowed to sink into the cornea to estimate IOP. The number of weights on the probe correlates with an IOP determined by a conversion chart provided by the device. Schwartz et al found that, on average, Schiotz underestimated GAT by 1.1 mm Hg. This device is not commonly used today given the need for supine position, corneal anesthesia, and creation of easier-to-use devices.[24]

NONCONTACT OR AIR-PUFF TONOMETRY

Created by Dr. Bernard Grolman in the 1950s, the air-puff tonometer determines IOP by measuring the time necessary for a given force of air to flatten a certain area of the cornea. When the air contacts the cornea, an infrared light beam is reflected off the flattened surface. The amount of light reflected is compared with time of applanation, allowing an estimation of IOP. The noncontact tonometer is simple to use, requires minimal training, and has no risk of infection transmission. Older versions of the air-puff tonometer had a ± 3 mm Hg difference as compared to GAT and tended to overestimate lower IOP and underestimate higher IOP. However, modern versions correlate well with GAT, overestimating IOP by only 0.12 to 0.58 mm Hg.[25-28]

OCULAR RESPONSE ANALYZER

The ORA is a noncontact tonometer that uses an air jet to apply force to the cornea and an electro-optical system to determine the IOP. As the cornea moves inward and outward in response to the increasing and decreasing velocity of the air jet, its deformation is tracked. The instrument makes 2 measurements: the force required to flatten the cornea as the air pressure rises, and the force at which the cornea flattens again as the air pressure falls. The difference between the 2 measurements is termed *corneal hysteresis* (CH). The average of air pressure rising and air pressure falling provides a Goldmann-correlated IOP value. In addition to these 2 values, ORA also provides a corneal-compensated IOP, which takes corneal biomechanical properties into account.[29-35]

DIGITAL TONOMETRY

It is possible to estimate IOP by digital pressure on the globe, referred to as *palpation* or *digital tonometry*. This method may be inaccurate even in very experienced hands and is useful only for detecting large differences between the patient's 2 eyes.

TRANSPALPEBRAL TONOMETRY

Transpalpebral tonometry measures IOP through the eyelid. One such device, the Diaton (BiCOM Inc), measures IOP by measuring the rebound of a free-falling rod against the tarsal plate of the eyelid overlying the sclera. It is not used in routine clinical practice, as it has poor agreement with GAT.[36]

FACTORS THAT AFFECT INTRAOCULAR PRESSURE MEASUREMENTS

Aside from surface tension and corneal parameters that can affect IOP measurements, there are also other factors that should be considered that impact the measured pressure regardless of technique (Table 3-1). CCT has been shown to be an independent risk factor for the development of glaucoma and should be checked in every patient who is being evaluated for glaucoma. Patients with thinner CCT tend to have underestimations of their IOP, while patients with thicker CCT tend to have overestimated IOP.[37]

CH has been shown to be an important inherent characteristic of the cornea that can influence eye pressure measurements. Patients with lower CH tend to have higher IOP readings, and patients with higher CH tend to have lower IOP readings. Furthermore, low CH has been shown to be predictive of visual field progression.[38] In a study of glaucomatous eyes, ORA corneal-compensated IOP showed a greater correlation with visual field loss than IOP measured by rebound tonometry or with GAT.[39]

In general, when a cornea is altered from its natural state, there is a potential for artifacts with IOP measurement. Eyes with prior incisional refractive surgery or incisional corneal surgery demonstrate lower CH and higher corneal corrected IOP.[40] In edematous cadaveric eyes, it was found that Tono-Pen and iCare pressures underestimate pressures with Tono-Pen pressure being closer to true pressure.[41]

Table 3-1. Factors That Influence Intraocular Pressure Readings

OCULAR FACTORS	NON-OCULAR FACTORS
Corneal thickness	Body habitus of patient
Corneal hysteresis	Patient clothing (neck tie, tight collar)
Corneal astigmatism	Patient holding breath
Prior corneal surgery	Valsalva maneuver
Corneal scar	External pressure placed on ocular adnexa by examiner
Corneal edema	Calibration of machine

Artifacts can also occur during measurement. Patient straining or squeezing or accidental pressure on the globe by the examiner can lead to false overestimation of IOP. Corneal astigmatism can lead to errors in readings; thus, 2 measurements 90 degrees apart is usually recommended. Limitation in episcleral venous flow, such as from increased intrathoracic pressure, a necktie, or tight-fitting clothes, could lead to falsely overestimated IOP. It is important to be mindful of these situations.

THE FUTURE OF MEASURING INTRAOCULAR PRESSURE

Diurnal variation in IOP is an important factor to consider when interpreting stability of disease. Solely obtaining IOP readings during routine office visits can limit the clinician's understanding of how IOP fluctuation may be causing progression of a patient's disease. New home monitoring, continuous monitoring, and implantable monitoring devices are currently in development and may be of great use in the management of this disease.

There are 3 main categories of 24-hour IOP monitoring devices that are currently available or in development: self-monitoring, temporary continuous monitoring, and permanent continuous monitoring.[42] Self-monitoring devices, such as the Tono-Pen and the iCare, have already been discussed above.

Sensimed has introduced the Triggerfish contact lens sensor, which is currently approved in Europe and has recently been approved by the US Food and Drug Administration. The contact lens sensor is a soft, disposable silicone contact lens embedding a microsensor that captures spontaneous circumferential changes at the corneoscleral area. An embedded microprocessor transmits an output signal to an adhesive wireless antenna that is secured externally to the periocular surface. The wireless antenna recharges the microprocessor and simultaneously receives continuous data, which is transferred by a cable wire to a portable recorder worn at the patient's side that allows the patient to be ambulatory.[43]

The Implandata EyeMate (permanent continuous monitoring) is a wireless intraocular transducer that consists of 8 pressure sensors and is compatible with ciliary sulcus placement. Each pressure sensor is composed of 2 parallel plates, and as the distance between the 2 plates varies with changes in IOP, a signal is generated that is transmitted to a hand-held reader unit.[44]

CONCLUSION

Accurate and precise IOP measurements are essential to the clinical and surgical management of glaucoma. Currently, there are many devices that can be used depending on the clinical setting. New devices are being created to monitor IOP at several time points throughout the day to better understand diurnal fluctuation of IOP on progression of disease.

REFERENCES

1. Kass MA, Heuer DK, Higginbotham EJ, et al. The Ocular Hypertension Treatment Study: a randomized trial determines that topical ocular hypotensive medication delays or prevents the onset of primary open-angle glaucoma. *Arch Ophthalmol.* 2002;120:701-713.
2. Heijl A, Leske MC, Bengtsoon B, et al. Early Manifest Glaucoma Trial Group. Reduction of intraocular pressure and glaucoma progression: results from the Early Manifest Glaucoma Trial. *Arch Ophthalmol.* 2002;120:1268-1279.
3. Lichter PR, Musch DC, Gillespie BW, et al. Interim clinical outcomes in the Collaborative Initial Glaucoma Treatment Study comparing initial treatment randomized to medication or surgery. *Ophthalmology.* 2001;108:1943-1953.
4. De Moraes CGV, Prata TS, Liebmann J, Ritch R. Modalities of tonometry and their accuracy with respect to corneal thickness and irregularities. *J Optom.* 2008;1(2):43-49. doi:10.3921/joptom.2008.43
5. Wozniak K, Köller AU, Spörl E. Intraocular pressure measurement during the day and night for glaucoma patients and normal controls using Goldmann and Perkins applanation tonometry. *Ophthalmologe.* 2006;103:1027-1031.
6. Baskett JS, Goen TM, Terry JE. A comparison of Perkins and Goldmann applanation tonometry. *J Am Optom Assoc.* 1986;57:832-834.
7. Azuara-Blanco A, Bhojani TK, Sarhan AR. Tono-pen determination of intraocular pressure in patients with band keratopathy or glued cornea. *Br J Ophthalmol.* 1998;82:634-636.
8. Salvetat ML, Zeppieri M, Tosoni C. Comparisons between Pascal dynamic contour tonometry, the TonoPen, and Goldmann applanation tonometry in patients with glaucoma. *Acta Ophthalmol Scand.* 2007;85:272-279.
9. Broman AT, Congdon NG, Bandeen-Roche K. Influence of corneal structure, corneal responsiveness, and other ocular parameters on tonometric measurement of intraocular pressure. *J Glaucoma.* 2007;16:581-588.
10. Ceruti P, Morbio R, Marraffa M, Marchini G. Comparison of Goldmann applanation tonometry and dynamic contour tonometry in healthy and glaucomatous eyes. *Eye.* 2008:25.
11. Schneider E, Grehn F. Intraocular pressure measurement-comparison of dynamic contour tonometry and Goldmann applanation tonometry. *J Glaucoma.* 2006;15:2-6.
12. Fresco BB. A new tonometer—the pressure phosphene tonometer: clinical comparison with Goldman tonometry. *Ophthalmology.* 1998;105:2123-2126.
13. Papastergiou GI, Kozobolis V, Siganos DS. Assessment of the pascal dynamic contour tonometer in measuring intraocular pressure in keratoconic eyes. *J Glaucoma.* 2008;17:484-488.

14. Meyenberg A, Iliev ME, Eschmann R, Frueh BE. Dynamic contour tonometry in keratoconus and postkeratoplasty eyes. *Cornea.* 2008;27:305-310.

15. Barreto J, Jr, Babic M, Vessani RM. Dynamic contour tonometry and Goldman applanation tonometry in eyes with keratoconus. *Clinics.* 2006;61:511-514.

16. Hamilton KE, Pye DC, Kao L. The effect of corneal edema on dynamic contour and goldmann tonometry. *Optom Vis Sci.* 2008;85:451-456.

17. Viestenz A, Langenbucher A, Seitz B. Evaluation of dynamic contour tonometry in penetrating keratoplasties. *Ophthalmologe.* 2006;103:773-776.

18. Van der Jagt LH, Jansonius NM. Three portable tonometers, the TGDc-01, the ICARE and the Tonopen XL, compared with each other and with Goldmann applanation tonometry. *Ophthalmic Physiol Opt.* 2005;25:429-435.

19. Chui WS, Lam A, Chen D. The influence of corneal properties on rebound tonometry. *Ophthalmology.* 2008;115:80-84.

20. Jóhannesson G, Hallberg P, Eklund A. Pascal, ICare and Goldmann applanation tonometry—a comparative study. *Acta Ophthalmol.* 2008;86:614-621.

21. Brusini P, Salvetat ML, Zeppieri M. Comparison of ICare tonometer with Goldmann applanation tonometer in glaucoma patients. *J Glaucoma.* 2006;15:213-217.

22. Fernandes P, Díaz-Rey JA, Queirós A. Comparison of the ICare rebound tonometer with the Goldmann tonometer in a normal population. *Ophthalmic Physiol Opt.* 2005;25:436-440.

23. Tonnu PA, Ho T, Sharma K. A comparison of four methods of tonometry: method agreement and interobserver variability. *Br J Ophthalmol.* 2005;89:847-850.

24. Schwartz JT, Dell'Osso GG. Comparison of Goldmann and Schiotz tonometry in a community. *Arch Ophthalmol.* 1966;75(6):788-795.

25. Moseley MJ, Evans NM, Fielder AR. Comparison of a new non-contact tonometer with Goldmann applanation. *Eye.* 1989;3:332-337.

26. Gupta V, Sony P, Agarwal HC. Inter-instrument agreement and influence of central corneal thickness on measurements with Goldmann, pneumotonometer and noncontact tonometer in glaucomatous eyes. *Indian J Ophthalmol.* 2006;54:261-265.

27. Parker VA., Herrtage J, Sarkies NJ. Clinical comparison of the Keeler Pulsair 3000 with Goldmann applanation tonometry. *Br J Ophthalmol.* 2001;85:1303-1304.

28. Jorge J, Díaz-Rey JA, González-Méijome JM. Clinical performance of the Reichert AT550: a new non-contact tonometer. *Ophthalmic Physiol Opt.* 2002;22:560-564.

29. Sullivan-Mee M, Billingsley SC, Patel AD. Ocular response analyzer in subjects with and without glaucoma. *Optom Vis Sci.* 2008;85:463-470.

30. Laiquzzaman M, Bhojwani R. Cunliffe Diurnal variation of ocular hysteresis in normal subjects: relevance in clinical context. *Clin Experiment Ophthalmol.* 2006;34:114-118.

31. Touboul D, Roberts C, Kérautret J. Correlations between corneal hysteresis, intraocular pressure, and corneal central pachymetry. *J Cataract Refract Surg.* 2008;34:616-622.

32. Lim LS, Gazzard G, Chan YH. Cornea biomechanical characteristics and their correlates with refractive error in Singapore children. *Invest Ophthalmol Vis Sci.* 2008;49:3852-3857.

33. Kynigopoulos M, Schlote T, Kotecha A. Repeatability of intraocular pressure and corneal biomechanical properties measurements by the ocular response analyzer. *Klin Monatsbl Augenheilkd.* 2008;225:357-360.

34. Hager A, Schroeder B, Sadeghi M. The influence of corneal hysteresis and corneal resistance factor on the measurement of intraocular pressure. *Ophthalmologe.* 2007;104:484-489.

35. Annette H, Kristina L, Bernd S. Effect of central corneal thickness and corneal hysteresis on tonometry as measured by dynamic contour tonometry, ocular response analyzer, and Goldmann tonometry in glaucomatous eyes. *J Glaucoma.* 2008;17:361-365.

36. Doherty MD, Carrim ZI, O'Neill DP. Diaton tonometry: an assessment of validity and preference against Goldmann tonometry. *Clin Exp Ophthalmol.* 2012;40(4):e171-e175. doi:10.1111/j.1442-9071.2011.02636.x

37. Brandt JD. Central corneal thickness, tonometry, and glaucoma risk- a guide for the perplexed. *Can J Ophthalmol.* 2007;42(4):562-566.

38. Congdon NG, Broman AT, Bandeen-Roche, Grover D, Quigley HA. Central corneal thickness and corneal hysteresis associated with glaucoma damage. *Am J Ophthalmol.* 2016;141(5):868-875.

39. Susanna BN, Ogata NG, Daga FB, et al. Association between rates of visual field progression and intraocular pressure measurements obtained by different tonometers. *Ophthalmology.* 2019;126(1):49-54.

40. Hardin JS, Lee CI, Lane LF, Hester CC, Morshedi RG. Corneal hysteresis in post-radial keratotomy primary open-angle glaucoma. *Graefes Arch Clin Exp Ophthalmol.* 2018;256(10):1971-1976.

41. Ruland K, Olanyanju J, Borras T, Grewal DS, Fleischman D. Accuracy of tonopen vs. iCare in human cadaveric eyes with edematous corneas over a wide range of intraocular pressure. *J Glaucoma.* 2019;28(5):e82-e85. doi:10.1097/IJG.0000000000001162

42. Morales-Fernandez L, Garcia-Bella J, Martinez-de-la-Casa JM, et al. Changes in corneal biomechanical properties after 24 hours of continuous intraocular pressure monitoring using a contact lens sensor. *Can J Ophthalmol.* 2018;53(3):236-241.

43. Sensimed, Inc. Sensimed triggerfish. https://www.sensimed.ch/sensimed-triggerfish/. Accessed January 29, 2019.

44. IOP: Implandata ophthalmic products GmbH. http://implandata.com/en/. Accessed January 29, 2019.

4

Anterior Segment Imaging
What Should You Use and When?

Janice Kim, MD; Kitiya Ratanawongphaibul, MD;
and Teresa C. Chen, MD

INTRODUCTION

Gonioscopy has been the gold standard for evaluating the angle. However, gonioscopy can be limited by subjective evaluation, indentation error, operator experience, varying lighting conditions, and uncooperative patients.[1-4] As technology has advanced, anterior segment imaging has become a valuable adjunctive tool, not only for diagnosing lesions posterior to the iris, but also for elucidating underlying structural mechanisms for outflow resistance.

Ultrasound biomicroscopy (UBM) and anterior segment optical coherence tomography (AS-OCT) are the 2 most common anterior segment imaging modalities used today. Both allow for objective quantitative cross-sectional imaging of the anterior chamber angle, and both provide high-resolution reproducible images in both light and dark conditions.[5,6] This chapter will discuss the general principles of UBM and AS-OCT and their associated clinical applications in glaucoma (Table 4-1).

Panarelli JF, ed.
The Pocket Guide to Glaucoma (pp 39-55).
© 2022 Taylor & Francis Group.

Table 4-1. Summary

ANTERIOR SEGMENT IMAGING MODALITY	ADVANTAGES	DISADVANTAGES	MAIN CLINICAL APPLICATIONS
UBM	• Can image structures posterior to iris, such as the ciliary body • Can image in the presence of cloudy or opaque media	• Direct contact method, with associated patient discomfort, corneal abrasion and infection risk, and inadvertent angle distortion secondary to indentation • Time-consuming • Requires skilled operator • Smaller field of view	• Identify angle-closure pathologies, such as plateau iris syndrome and iridociliary cysts and tumors • Imaging the presence and extent of cyclodialysis clefts

(continued)

Table 4-1. Summary (continued)			
ANTERIOR SEGMENT IMAGING MODALITY	ADVANTAGES	DISADVANTAGES	MAIN CLINICAL APPLICATIONS
AS-OCT	• Noncontact method, allowing immediate postoperative use and anterior segment imaging without inadvertent distortion • Rapid image acquisition • Does not require a skilled operator • High axial resolution • Wider field of view	• Expensive • Cannot image structures behind the iris • Difficulty imaging through media opacities	• Postoperative evaluation of filtering blebs and glaucoma surgical implants (ie, MIGS devices) • Detecting corneal fluid interfaces after LASIK procedures

AS-OCT = anterior segment optical coherence tomography; MIGS = minimally invasive glaucoma surgery; UBM = ultrasound biomicroscopy.

ULTRASOUND BIOMICROSCOPY

Ultrasound Technology Principles

UBM is a high-resolution ultrasound technique providing in vivo B-scan images of the anterior segment. To create the images, the UBM transducer transmits sound waves with frequencies ranging from 35 to 100 MHz, and images are created due to the varying echogenicity of different ocular tissue interface densities.[1,2,4,6] The transducer frequency impacts the depth of penetration and tissue resolution for ultrasonography.[7] In contrast to conventional B-scan ultrasonography with transducer frequencies ranging from 7.5 to 10 MHz, the UBM transducer frequency is around 50 MHz, which provides higher image resolutions of about 20 μm axially and 40 to 50 μm laterally and tissue depth penetration of up to 4 to 5 mm.[2,4,6-9]

Advantages of Ultrasound Biomicroscopy

UBM has some advantages over AS-OCT, such as greater depth of tissue penetration. For example, unlike AS-OCT, UBM can image behind the iris to better visualize structures, such as the ciliary body, the sulcus space, the zonules, the anterior lens capsule, and the anterior choroid (Figure 4-1A).[2,4-10] On UBM, the scleral spur—the region where the radio-opaque shadow of the sclera merges with the radiolucent shadow of the cornea—is the reference point used to identify these ocular structures (see Figure 4-1A).[5,7,8] Compared to AS-OCT, UBM is better for examining cysts and tumors behind the iris, for determining if the suspected lesion is solid or cystic, for measuring the full extent of the lesion, and for determining progression or regression of the lesion size.[8,9] Unlike AS-OCT, which utilizes a light source, UBM can better image anterior chamber structures through an opacified cornea.[4] For all these reasons, UBM has the ability to elucidate etiologies for angle closure,[6] such as plateau iris, ciliary body cysts, and anterior segment tumors.

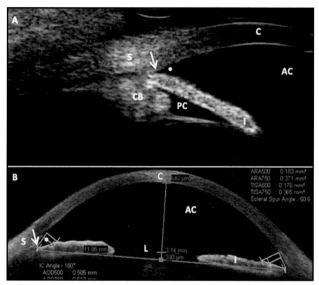

Figure 4-1. Normal anterior segment anatomy on (A) UBM and (B) AS-OCT depicting the scleral spur (white arrow) as well as the cornea (C), anterior chamber (AC), iris (I), posterior chamber (PC), lens (L), sclera (S), ciliary body (CB), and anterior chamber angle (asterisk). The AS-OCT image also depicts the angle-opening distance (AOD; perpendicular distance between a point 500 or 750 μm [AOD 500 or 750] from the scleral spur to the opposing iris), angle recess area (triangular area 500 or 750 μm from the scleral spur [angle recess area 500 or 750] bounded by the AOD, the anterior iris surface and the inner corneoscleral wall), and the trabecular iris space area (trapezoidal area 500 or 750 μm [trabecular iris space area 500 or 750] from the scleral spur bounded by the AOD, the anterior iris surface, the inner corneoscleral wall, and the perpendicular distance between the scleral spur and the opposing iris). (Reproduced with permission from Alexis LaVerde, CDOS.)

Limitations of Ultrasound Biomicroscopy

UBM is not without its own set of limitations. For example, UBM requires a coupling medium, which is uncomfortable for the patient since it directly contacts the eye and can introduce risks of corneal abrasion and infection.[2] Another issue is that patients are supine position during scanning, which may theoretically alter the anterior chamber depth and angle opening by causing the iris diaphragm to fall back.[6] Ultimately, the main limitation of UBM results from its difficulty in acquiring images, which is impacted by probe alignment and consistent patient fixation.[4] Therefore, compared to AS-OCT, UBM can be more time-consuming and requires a skilled operator to obtain precise high-quality images.[1,6]

Clinical Applications of Ultrasound Biomicroscopy for Glaucoma Evaluation

Determining Etiologies of Angle Closure

- **Plateau iris configuration:** UBM can confirm a clinical diagnosis of plateau iris. The classic plateau iris UBM finding is anteriorly positioned ciliary processes that push the peripheral iris up toward the angle.[3,10] This results in a steep rise in the peripheral iris, with a relatively flat iris plane elsewhere; and this also results in closure of the sulcus between the iris and ciliary body (Figure 4-2).[1,5,6,8,10,11]

- **Iridociliary lesions:** UBM is useful for detecting iris and ciliary body lesions and for distinguishing cysts from solid tumors of the iris and ciliary body. UBM enables visualization of angle narrowing due to cysts (Figure 4-3A) or tumors (Figure 4-3B).[2]

- Specifically, UBM can be used to see the following iridociliary lesions:

  ○ **Iris cysts:** UBM can detect iris cysts, such as iris pigment epithelial cysts, congenital iris stromal cysts, parasitic cysts, secondary cysts from trauma or surgical procedures (ie, conjunctival or corneal epithelial downgrowth), drug-induced iris cysts secondary to miotics or latanoprost, or cysts secondary to intraocular tumors, such as medulloepitheliomas, uveal melanomas, and uveal nevi.[12]

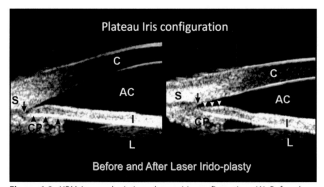

Figure 4-2. UBM image depicting plateau iris configuration. (A) Before laser iridoplasty. The image shows the ciliary body (CB) contacting the posterior iris (black arrowheads), placing the peripheral iris in opposition to the trabecular meshwork. The CB normally does not touch the posterior iris. (B) After laser iridoplasty. The image shows the opening of the anterior chamber angle (white arrowheads) after iridoplasty. The cornea (C), anterior chamber (AC), iris (I), lens (L), ciliary sulcus (CP), and scleral spur (S; black arrow) are visible. (Reproduced with permission from Salim S, Dorairaj S. Anterior segment imaging in glaucoma. *Semin Ophthalmol.* 2013;28[3]:113-125. www.tandfonline.com)

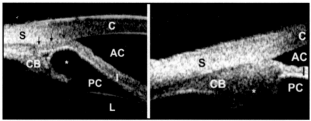

Figure 4-3. UBM image depicting (A) angle closure due to an iridociliary cyst (asterisk) and (B) an iridociliary tumor (asterisk). (A) The image shows the iris root being pushed toward the cornea, resulting in total angle occlusion (arrows). (B) The ciliary body is abnormally large involving the iris root and pars plana. The cornea (C), anterior chamber (AC), iris (I), posterior chamber (PC), lens (L), ciliary body (CB), and sclera (S) are visible. (Reproduced from Ishikawa H, Schuman JS. Anterior segment imaging: ultrasound biomicroscopy. *Ophthalmol Clin North Am.* 2004;17[1]:7-20, with permission from Elsevier.)

- ○ **Iris tumors:** UBM can image iris tumors, such as nevi,[13] melanomas, medulloepitheliomas, leiomyomas,[14] melanocytomas, adenomas of the iris pigment epithelium,[12] hemangiomas,[15] iris plasmacytomas,[16] and metastatic tumors[17] (ie, from conjunctival squamous cell carcinoma,[18] renal cell carcinomas,[19] small and large cell carcinomas of the lung,[20-22] lymphomas,[23] and prostate carcinomas[24,25]).

- ○ **Ciliary body cysts:** UBM is particularly helpful for localizing ciliary body cysts, which can occur in the pars plicata or the pars plana of the ciliary body.[26] These cysts include congenital cysts[27] and ciliary epithelial cysts.[28] Like iris cysts, secondary cysts of the ciliary body can also be from trauma or surgical procedures (ie, epithelial downgrowth)[29] and drugs, such as miotics or latanoprost.[30]

- ○ **Ciliary body tumors:** Ciliary body tumors that can be imaged with UBM include nevi,[31,32] malignant melanomas, melanocytomas,[33] and rarer tumors, such as leiomyomas,[34] medulloepitheliomas,[35] adenomas (ie, coronal adenomas),[36] adenocarcinomas,[31,37] intraocular tumor invasion (ie, conjunctival squamous cell carcinoma),[18] ciliary body oligodendrogliomas,[38] ciliary body schwannomas,[39,40] and hemangiomas.[41]

- • **Malignant glaucoma (or aqueous misdirection):** Malignant glaucoma is a rare postoperative complication of which the mechanism is not fully understood. Some believe it is the result of aqueous being diverted into the posterior segment, possibly due to an anatomical change in the relationship between the ciliary body, anterior hyaloid face, and vitreous body.[42] Another school of thought revolves around choroidal expansion as the primary mechanism. These posterior forces push the iris-lens diaphragm forward, leading to a uniformly shallow anterior chamber.[1,8,10] UBM may help distinguish malignant glaucoma from pupillary block glaucoma, as it can more clearly demonstrate the central and peripheral axial shallowing characteristic of this process.[42-44]

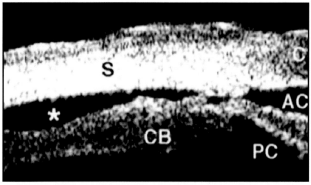

Figure 4-4. UBM image depicting a cyclodialysis cleft. The ciliary body (CB) is avulsed from the sclera (S), resulting in free aqueous flow from the anterior chamber (AC) through the cleft into the supraciliary space (asterisk). The cornea (C) and posterior chamber (PC) are visible. (Reproduced from Ishikawa H, Schuman JS. Anterior segment imaging: ultrasound biomicroscopy. *Ophthalmol Clin North Am.* 2004;17[1]:7-20, with permission from Elsevier.)

Blunt Ocular Trauma

- **Cyclodialysis clefts:** Blunt ocular trauma can cause cyclodialysis clefts, which occurs when the ciliary body detaches from the scleral spur to create an abnormal drainage pathway that may lead to hypotony.[45] UBM is useful in cases where the cleft is not visible on gonioscopy. It is also particularly valuable for detecting the presence and extent of cyclodialysis clefts, especially if visualization is limited by opacities such as hyphemas or by abnormal anterior segment morphology.[3,5,7,8,10] Clefts on UBM can be seen as a black hypoechoic communication between the anterior chamber and the suprachoroidal space (Figure 4-4).[46]

ANTERIOR SEGMENT
OPTICAL COHERENCE TOMOGRAPHY

Optical Coherence Tomography Technology Principles

AS-OCT is a high-resolution 3-dimensional imaging modality that utilizes the differing light reflectivity of different ocular tissues to create a cross-sectional image of the eye from the cornea to the iris.[4,47,48] To create 3-dimensional images, the OCT machine emits a low-coherence infrared light via a beam splitter into 2 directions (ie, to a reference arm and to the eye) and then measures the time delay between light backscattered from the reference arm and from ocular tissues.[48,49] The OCT then superimposes the reflected light signals from each arm at an interferometer to create an interference pattern, which is converted to an electrical signal.[48-52] The strength of each electrical signal is then converted into depth information for an axial scan. The OCT then combines a series of these axial scans to produce the final 2-dimensional or 3-dimensional map of the various tissue structures.[49,50,53]

Current AS-OCT machines use either spectral-domain OCT (SD-OCT) or swept-source OCT (SS-OCT) technologies, which have different light source properties. SD-OCT generally utilizes a broad bandwidth laser source with a spectrometer, and SS-OCT may use a monochromatic laser source with a photodetector in order to detect the interference signal.[48] Additionally, the central median wavelength for SS-OCT (1050 nm) is longer than that for SD-OCT (840 nm), which allows SS-OCT to more deeply penetrate the iris and sclera.[3,48,54] Axial resolutions for SD-OCT and SS-OCT are similar at 4 to 7 μm, while imaging speeds are faster for SS-OCT compared to SD-OCT.[3]

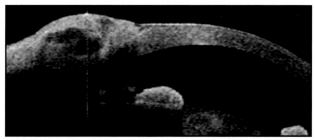

Figure 4-5. AS-OCT image depicting a functioning bleb after trabeculectomy. (Reproduced with permission from Salim S, Dorairaj S. Anterior segment imaging in glaucoma. *Semin Ophthalmol*. 2013;28[3]:113-125. www.tandfonline.com)

Advantages of Anterior Segment Optical Coherence Tomography

AS-OCT has several advantages over UBM. For one, AS-OCT imaging has better axial resolution (Figure 4-1B) and faster sampling rates, while imaging the entire cross-section of the eye at a greater working distance. Secondly, AS-OCT scans patients in a seated, upright position and is noncontact and nonoperator dependent, which makes these scans more comfortable for patients and avoids artifacts from inadvertent corneal indentation.[6,53,55] This also makes AS-OCT particularly useful for assessing post-trabeculectomy blebs (Figure 4-5) due to the noncontact nature of the test, minimizing bleb trauma and potential infections.[6,56]

Limitations of Anterior Segment Optical Coherence Tomography

A major disadvantage of AS-OCT is its inability to visualize deeper ocular structures behind the iris since infrared light cannot penetrate beyond the iris posterior pigmented epithelium, limiting visualization of the ciliary body and other posterior structures.[2,50,52] Additionally, unlike UBM, AS-OCT's light source has difficulty imaging through opaque media or through eyelids to image the superior and inferior angles.[52,57]

Clinical Applications of Anterior Segment Optical Coherence Tomography in Glaucoma

Postoperative Imaging

- **Imaging bleb morphology:** A filtering bleb allows for both the aqueous outflow to the bleb and its absorption through conjunctival vessels around the bleb.[9] AS-OCT can visualize bleb walls, intrableb cysts, wall thickness, and bleb dimensions. In certain cases, suboptimal bleb function can be predicted based on the bleb morphology (see Figure 4-5).[9] When imaged with AS-OCT, well-functioning blebs will tend to have a large internal fluid-filled cavity, extensive hyporeflective area, and thicker bleb walls with numerous microcysts.[52] AS-OCT can also be used to image implants used to facilitate outflow in glaucoma surgery, such as the Xen Gel Stent (Allergan) or the Ologen matrix (Aeon Astron Europe B.V.), a biodegradable porcine derived implant.[55,58]

- **Imaging minimally invasive glaucoma surgery (MIGS):** MIGS aims to reduce intraocular pressure in a safer, less invasive way than through traditional trabeculectomy surgery. MIGS procedures often use implants aimed at increasing trabecular outflow (eg, iStent [Glaukos]; Hydrus Microstent [Ivantis]) or subconjunctival filtration (eg, Xen Gel Stent). AS-OCT can confirm proper implant placement as well as assess bleb morphology during follow-up.[59,60]

- **Glaucoma imaging after LASIK:** AS-OCT visualization of a fluid interface between the stromal bed and the LASIK flap is critical (Figure 4-6)[61,62] because the fluid interface can cause artifactually low Goldmann applanation tonometry readings. This interface fluid can develop after LASIK due to transudation of aqueous fluid through the corneal endothelium and into the flap interface. This LASIK-flap associated complication is thought to arise from a high intraocular pressure gradient caused by steroid use postoperatively.

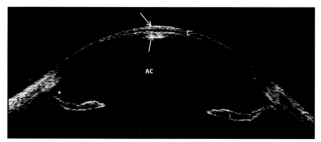

Figure 4-6. AS-OCT can detect a fluid interface (arrows) between the stromal bed and the LASIK flap of the cornea (C). The anterior chamber (AC), iris (I), sclera (S), and anterior chamber angle (asterisk) are also visible. (Reproduced with permission from Milica Margeta, MD, PhD.)

Calculating Central Corneal Thickness

Central corneal thickness (CCT) is essential in any glaucoma evaluation. Although ultrasound pachymetry is the gold standard for measuring CCT, AS-OCT is another favorable noninvasive, high-resolution imaging method for measuring CCT with measurements comparable to ultrasound pachymetry.[63,64]

ACKNOWLEDGMENTS

Teresa C. Chen's research is supported in part by the Fidelity Charitable fund.

REFERENCES

1. Ursea R, Silverman RH. Anterior-segment imaging for assessment of glaucoma. *Expert Rev Ophthalmol.* 2010;5(1):59-74. doi:10.1586/eop.09.61
2. See JLS. Imaging of the anterior segment in glaucoma. *Clin Experiment Ophthalmol.* 2009;37(5):506-513. doi:10.1111/j.1442-9071.2009.02081.x
3. Maslin JS, Barkana Y, Dorairaj SK. Anterior segment imaging in glaucoma: an updated review. *Indian J Ophthalmol.* 2015;63(8):630-640. doi:10.4103/0301-4738.169787

4. Blieden LS. Diagnostic Imaging of the anterior segment in glaucoma: an update. *Int Ophthalmol Clin.* 2017;57(3):125-136. doi:10.1097/IIO.0000000000000173

5. Nolan W. Anterior segment imaging: ultrasound biomicroscopy and anterior segment optical coherence tomography. *Curr Opin Ophthalmol.* 2008;19(2):115-121. doi:10.1097/ICU.0b013e3282f40bba

6. Salim S, Dorairaj S. Anterior segment imaging in glaucoma. *Semin Ophthalmol.* 2013;28(3):113-125. doi:10.3109/08820538.2013.777749

7. Liebmann JM. Ultrasound biomicroscopy of the anterior segment. *J Glaucoma.* 2001;10(5 Suppl 1):S53-S55.

8. Dada T, Gadia R, Sharma A, et al. Ultrasound biomicroscopy in glaucoma. *Surv Ophthalmol.* 2011;56(5):433-450. doi:10.1016/j.survophthal.2011.04.004

9. Golez E, Latina M. The use of anterior segment imaging after trabeculectomy. *Semin Ophthalmol.* 2012;27(5-6):155-159. doi:10.3109/08820538.2012.707275

10. Ishikawa H, Schuman JS. Anterior segment imaging: ultrasound biomicroscopy. *Ophthalmol Clin N Am.* 2004;17(1):7-20. doi:10.1016/j.ohc.2003.12.001

11. Stefan C, Iliescu DA, Batras M, Timaru CM, De Simone A. plateau iris—diagnosis and treatment. *Romanian J Ophthalmol.* 2015;59(1):14-18.

12. Georgalas I, Petrou P, Papaconstantinou D, et al. Iris cysts: a comprehensive review on diagnosis and treatment. *Surv Ophthalmol.* 2018;63(3):347-364. doi:10.1016/j.survophthal.2017.08.009

13. Schwab C, Zalaudek I, Mayer C, et al. New insights into oculodermal nevogenesis and proposal for a new iris nevus classification. *Br J Ophthalmol.* 2015;99(5):644-649. doi:10.1136/bjophthalmol-2014-305849

14. Benarous A, Sevestre H, Drimbea A, Claisse A-S, Milazzo S. [Iris leiomyoma: a benign tumor in an atypical location]. *J Fr Ophtalmol.* 2015;38(2):e29-e32. doi:10.1016/j.jfo.2014.05.014

15. Shields JA, Bianciotto C, Kligman BE, Shields CL. Vascular tumors of the iris in 45 patients: the 2009 Helen Keller Lecture. *Arch Ophthalmol Chic Ill 1960.* 2010;128(9):1107-1113. doi:10.1001/archophthalmol.2010.188

16. Stacey AW, Lavric A, Thaung C, Siddiq S, Sagoo MS. Solitary iris plasmacytoma with anterior chamber crystalline deposits. *Cornea.* 2017;36(7):875-877. doi:10.1097/ICO.0000000000001222

17. Shields JA, Shields CL, Kiratli H, de Potter P. Metastatic tumors to the iris in 40 patients. *Am J Ophthalmol.* 1995;119(4):422-430.

18. Gündüz K, Hosal BM, Zilelioglu G, Günalp I. The use of ultrasound biomicroscopy in the evaluation of anterior segment tumors and simulating conditions. *Ophthalmologica.* 2007;221(5):305-312. doi:10.1159/000104760

19. Portnoy SL, Arffa RC, Johnson BL, Terner IS. Metastatic renal cell carcinoma of the iris manifesting as an intrastromal iris cyst. *Am J Ophthalmol.* 1991;111(1):113-114.

20. Prause JU, Jensen OA, Eisgart F, Hansen U, Kieffer M. Bilateral diffuse malignant melanoma of the uvea associated with large cell carcinoma, giant cell type, of the lung. Case report of a newly described syndrome. *Ophthalmologica*. 1984;189(4):221-228. doi:10.1159/000309413

21. Hata M, Inoue T. Iris metastasis from small-cell lung cancer. *J Thorac Oncol Off Publ Int Assoc Study Lung Cancer*. 2014;9(10):1584-1585. doi:10.1097/JTO.0000000000000201

22. Karunanithi S, Sharma P, Jain S, Mukherjee A, Kumar R. Iris metastasis in a patient with small cell lung cancer: incidental detection with 18F-FDG PET/CT. *Clin Nucl Med*. 2014;39(6):554-555. doi:10.1097/RLU.0b013e3182a7549f

23. Mashayekhi A, Shields CL, Shields JA. Iris involvement by lymphoma: a review of 13 cases. *Clin Experiment Ophthalmol*. 2013;41(1):19-26. doi:10.1111/j.1442-9071.2012.02811.x

24. Martin V, Cuenca X, Lopez S, et al. Iris metastasis from prostate carcinoma: a case report and review of the literature. *Cancer Radiother J Soc Francaise Radiother Oncol*. 2015;19(5):331-333. doi:10.1016/j.canrad.2014.12.008

25. Mayama C, Ohashi M, Tomidokoro A, Kojima T. Bilateral iris metastases from prostate cancer. *Jpn J Ophthalmol*. 2003;47(1):69-71.

26. Allen RA, Miller DH, Straatsma BR. Cysts of the posterior ciliary body (pars plana). *Arch Ophthalmol Chic Ill 1960*. 1961;66:302-313.

27. Kunimatsu S, Araie M, Ohara K, Hamada C. Ultrasound biomicroscopy of ciliary body cysts. *Am J Ophthalmol*. 1999;127(1):48-55.

28. Davidson SI. Spontaneous cysts of the ciliary body. *Br J Ophthalmol*. 1960;44:461-466.

29. Taylor SJ. Case of implantation cyst of iris and ciliary body. *Br J Ophthalmol*. 1924;8(1):45-47.

30. Mohite AA, Prabhu RV, Ressiniotis T. Latanoprost induced iris pigment epithelial and ciliary body cyst formation in hypermetropic eyes. *Case Rep Ophthalmol Med*. 2017;2017:9362163. doi:10.1155/2017/9362163

31. Weisbrod DJ, Pavlin CJ, Emara K, et al. Small ciliary body tumors: ultrasound biomicroscopic assessment and follow-up of 42 patients. *Am J Ophthalmol*. 2006;141(4):622-628. doi:10.1016/j.ajo.2005.11.006

32. Taban M, Sears JE, Singh AD. Ciliary body naevus. *Eye Lond Engl*. 2007;21(12):1528-1530. doi:10.1038/sj.eye.6702622

33. Velazquez-Martin JP, Krema H, Fulda E, et al. Ultrasound biomicroscopy of the ciliary body in ocular/oculodermal melanocytosis. *Am J Ophthalmol*. 2013;155(4):681-687, 687.e1-2. doi:10.1016/j.ajo.2012.10.006

34. Croxatto JO, Malbran ES. Unusual ciliary body tumor. Mesectodermal leiomyoma. *Ophthalmology*. 1982;89(10):1208-1212.

35. Kaliki S, Shields CL, Eagle RC, et al. Ciliary body medulloepithelioma: analysis of 41 cases. *Ophthalmology*. 2013;120(12):2552-2559. doi:10.1016/j.ophtha.2013.05.015

36. Shields JA, Shields CL, Eagle RC, Friedman ES, Wheatley HM. Age-related hyperplasia of the nonpigmented ciliary body epithelium (Fuchs adenoma) simulating a ciliary body malignant neoplasm. *Arch Ophthalmol Chic Ill 1960.* 2009;127(9):1224-1225. doi:10.1001/archophthalmol.2009.217

37. Shields JA, Eagle RC, Ferguson K, Shields CL. Tumors of the nonpigmented epithelium of the ciliary body: the Lorenz E. Zimmerman Tribute Lecture. *Retina Phila Pa.* 2015;35(5):957-965. doi:10.1097/IAE.0000000000000445

38. Guo Q, Hao J, Sun S bin, et al. Oligodendroglioma of the ciliary body: a unique case report and the review of literature. *BMC Cancer.* 2010;10:579. doi:10.1186/1471-2407-10-579

39. Goto H, Mori H, Shirato S, Usui M. Ciliary body schwannoma successfully treated by local resection. *Jpn J Ophthalmol.* 2006;50(6):543-546. doi:10.1007/s10384-006-0362-9

40. Kim IT, Chang SD. Ciliary body schwannoma. *Acta Ophthalmol Scand.* 1999;77(4):462-466.

41. Isola VM. Hemangioma of the ciliary body: a case report and review of the literature. *Ophthalmologica.* 1996;210(4):239-243. doi:10.1159/000310716

42. Tello C, Chi T, Shepps G, Liebmann J, Ritch R. Ultrasound biomicroscopy in pseudophakic malignant glaucoma. *Ophthalmology.* 1993;100(9):1330-1334.

43. Ruben S, Tsai J, Hitchings RA. Malignant glaucoma and its management. *Br J Ophthalmol.* 1997;81(2):163-167.

44. Shaffer RN, Hoskins HD. Ciliary block (malignant) glaucoma. *Ophthalmology.* 1978;85(3):215-221.

45. González-Martín-Moro J, Contreras-Martín I, Muñoz-Negrete FJ, Gómez-Sanz F, Zarallo-Gallardo J. Cyclodialysis: an update. *Int Ophthalmol.* 2017;37(2):441-457. doi:10.1007/s10792-016-0282-8

46. Shah VA, Majji AB. Ultrasound biomicroscopic documentation of traumatic cyclodialysis cleft closure with hypotony by medical therapy. *Eye Lond Engl.* 2004;18(8):857-858. doi:10.1038/sj.eye.6701331

47. Radhakrishnan S, Yarovoy D. Development in anterior segment imaging for glaucoma. *Curr Opin Ophthalmol.* 2014;25(2):98-103. doi:10.1097/ICU.0000000000000026

48. Ang M, Baskaran M, Werkmeister RM, et al. Anterior segment optical coherence tomography. *Prog Retin Eye Res.* 2018;66:132-156. doi:10.1016/j.preteyeres.2018.04.002

49. Huang D, Izatt JA. Physics and fundamentals of anterior segment optical coherence technology. In: *Anterior Segment Optical Coherence Technology.* 1st ed. SLACK Incorporated; 2008:1-9.

50. Sathyan P, Shilpa S, Anitha A. Optical coherence tomography in glaucoma. *J Curr Glaucoma Pract.* 2012;6(1):1-5. doi:10.5005/jp-journals-10008-1099

51. Ce Z, Chew PTK. Anterior segment imaging with anterior segment optical coherence tomography. In: *Ophthalmological Imaging and Applications.* 1st ed. CRC Press; 2017:299-314.

52. Sharma R, Sharma A, Arora T, et al. Application of anterior segment optical coherence tomography in glaucoma. *Surv Ophthalmol.* 2014;59(3):311-327. doi:10.1016/j.survophthal.2013.06.005

53. Li H, Jhanji V, Dorairaj S, et al. Anterior segment optical coherence tomography and its clinical applications in glaucoma. *J Curr Glaucoma Pract.* 2012;6(2):68-74. doi:10.5005/jp-journals-10008-1109

54. Kishi S. Impact of swept source optical coherence tomography on ophthalmology. *Taiwan J Ophthalmol.* 2016;6(2):58-68. doi:10.1016/j.tjo.2015.09.002

55. Wang D, Lin S. New developments in anterior segment optical coherence tomography for glaucoma. *Curr Opin Ophthalmol.* 2016;27(2):111-117. doi:10.1097/ICU.0000000000000243

56. Leung CK, Yick DW, Kwong YY, et al. Analysis of bleb morphology after trabeculectomy with Visante anterior segment optical coherence tomography. *Br J Ophthalmol.* 2007;91(3):340-344. doi:10.1136/bjo.2006.100321

57. Angmo D, Nongpiur ME, Sharma R, et al. Clinical utility of anterior segment swept-source optical coherence tomography in glaucoma. *Oman J Ophthalmol.* 2016;9(1):3-10. doi:10.4103/0974-620X.176093

58. Mastropasqua R, Fasanella V, Agnifili L, et al. Anterior segment optical coherence tomography imaging of conjunctival filtering blebs after glaucoma surgery. *BioMed Res Int.* 2014;2014. doi:10.1155/2014/610623

59. Richter GM, Coleman AL. Minimally invasive glaucoma surgery: current status and future prospects. *Clin Ophthalmol Auckl NZ.* 2016;10:189-206. doi:10.2147/OPTH.S80490

60. Fea AM, Spinetta R, Cannizzo PML, et al. Evaluation of bleb morphology and reduction in IOP and glaucoma medication following implantation of a novel gel stent. *J Ophthalmol.* 2017;2017:9364910. doi:10.1155/2017/9364910

61. Pan BX, Margeta MA. Elevated intraocular pressure in a young man with a history of laser-assisted in situ keratomileusis. *JAMA Ophthalmol.* January 2019. doi:10.1001/jamaophthalmol.2018.5430

62. Hamilton DR, Manche EE, Rich LF, Maloney RK. Steroid-induced glaucoma after laser in situ keratomileusis associated with interface fluid. *Ophthalmology.* 2002;109(4):659-665.

63. Ramesh PV, Jha KN, Srikanth K. Comparison of central corneal thickness using anterior segment optical coherence tomography versus ultrasound pachymetry. *J Clin Diagn Res JCDR.* 2017;11(8):NC08-NC11. doi:10.7860/JCDR/2017/25595.10420

64. Ayala M, Strandås R. Accuracy of optical coherence tomography (OCT) in pachymetry for glaucoma patients. *BMC Ophthalmol.* 2015;15. doi:10.1186/s12886-015-0116-x

5

Optic Nerve Head Imaging in Glaucoma

*Ravneet S. Rai, MD; Gadi Wollstein, MD;
and Joel S. Schuman, MD*

Imaging of the optic nerve head (ONH) plays an important role in the identification and staging of glaucoma. When used alongside intraocular pressure measurements and standard automated perimetry, ONH imaging provides invaluable insights into the structural changes that occur along the course of the disease.[1] Certain ONH parameters, such as cup-to-disc ratio, rim area, cup volume, and rim volume are of particular interest in the context of glaucoma. Retinal nerve fiber layer (RNFL) and macular thickness are also highly relevant in this regard.

STRUCTURAL CHANGES IN GLAUCOMA

The physical structure of the ONH undergoes a number of predictable changes over the course of glaucomatous disease. Typical changes include enlarged cupping (Figure 5-1), decreased rim area, and thinning of the RNFL in the peripapillary region. Studies have shown that ONH cupping and RNFL thinning can precede functional losses in vision by up to 6 years.[2,3] It has been

Panarelli JF, ed.
The Pocket Guide to Glaucoma (pp 57-72).
© 2022 Taylor & Francis Group.

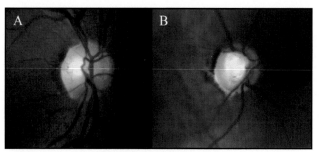

Figure 5-1. (A) Digital photograph of a normal disc. (B) Disc with enlarged cupping. The rim area is noticeably smaller compared to a normal disc, with localized thinning of the neuroretinal rim in the temporal, superior, and inferior regions.

estimated that between 25% and 35% of retinal ganglion cells are lost before visual field defects are detectable.[4] Several reasons have been proposed to explain this discrepancy. One reason is overlap in the receptive regions of adjacent ganglion cells primarily in the macula region, meaning that the area captured by damaged ganglion cells might be preserved by adjacent healthy cells.[5] Additionally, visual field threshold values are reported as logarithmic transformed values in order to reduce intersubject variability, especially between healthy individuals and early stages of glaucoma. This reduces the ability to detect early functional changes. It is also plausible that damage to structural integrity occurs first and only subsequently causes functional deficits.

The microvasculature in the peripapillary region also undergoes changes as glaucoma progresses. Healthy eyes have dense microvascular networks, while preperimetric glaucomatous eyes[6] and glaucomatous eyes[7] have been shown to have significantly diminished microvascular density.

Assessing changes in structural ONH parameters is important in identifying glaucoma and tracking its progression, particularly in early stages of the disease when functional losses have not yet occurred.[8] However, clinical examination is highly dependent on the clinician's skills and has high intersubject variability.[9] Considering that glaucoma causes irreversible neural damage, it is desirable to utilize the most sensitive and consistent means to detect changes. The introduction of imaging allows precise quantification and sensitive monitoring of tissue loss.[10] ONH imaging is also useful for detecting disease progression in late stages of glaucoma when other structural biomarkers reach their minimal measurable limit, known as the *floor effect*.[11] In caring for patients with glaucoma, the standard approach is to combine functional visual field testing with structural ONH imaging to get a full picture of the stage and rate of change of each individual's disease.

OPTIC NERVE HEAD IMAGING MODALITIES

Historically, imaging of the ONH was done using conventional film-based photography.[12] Since the integration of digital photography into the fundus camera in the late 1980s, clinicians have been able to quickly and easily capture high-resolution images of the optic disc. Evaluation of these images usually involves subjectively examining the cup-to-disc ratio and the neuroretinal rim area, important parameters in tracking glaucomatous progression.[12] Planimetry, a more quantitative approach, refers to a method of measuring disc size parameters from photographs while accounting for the magnification.[13] Glaucoma progression is usually slow, and identifying small changes in subsequent disc photography is clinically challenging. To mitigate this, image flickering registers the images and allows the user to flip between subsequent photographs, thus facilitating subjective detection of small changes.[14]

Disc photography can also reveal anomalies such as optic disc atrophy, optic disc drusen, disc hemorrhages, or peripapillary atrophy (Figure 5-2). Disc hemorrhages are linear hemorrhages oriented perpendicularly to the ONH.[15] In paitents with glaucoma, disc hemorrhages often co-localize with structural and functional damage and are often precursors for eventual glaucomatous damage.[15-17] However, because these hemorrhages tend to be absorbed within weeks to months, the clinical utility of this finding is limited.[18] Peripapillary atrophy is a finding that involves

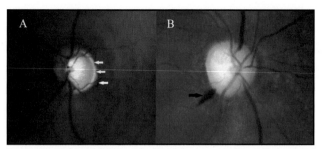

Figure 5-2. (A) Peripapillary atrophy. The yellow arrow indicates the border of the beta zone with exposed sclera, and the white arrow indicates the border of the more peripheral and pigmented alpha zone. (B) Disc hemorrhage located perpendicularly to the ONH (black arrow).

chorioretinal thinning and disturbance of the retinal pigment epithelium (RPE) in the region around the optic nerve.[19] While this finding can occur in benign conditions, it is also associated with glaucoma.[19] There is a spatial association between the location of chorioretinal thinning, sectors of optic nerve damage, and visual field loss.[20] Peripapillary atrophy has typically been classified into 2 zones: a peripheral alpha zone of structural irregularities in RPE cells, and a more central beta zone of chorioretinal thinning and loss of RPE cells with visible large choroidal vessels.[19] Recently, a gamma zone has also been described, which is a central area of parapapillary choroid that lacks overlying choroid, Bruch's membrane, and deep retinal layers.[21]

Moving beyond conventional photography, confocal scanning laser ophthalmoscopy (cSLO) is a technique that generates a 3-dimensional image of the ONH by using a diode laser to scan the retinal surface.[22] Without requiring pupil dilation, the scanning laser ophthalmoscope provides detailed visualization of the ONH region. By placing a pinhole, or confocal filter, in front of the detector, noise is reduced.[23] This allows for the acquisition of images with approximately 15 μm of transverse resolution and 300 μm axial resolution.[23] Once an image is acquired, the operator must mark the disc margin in order for the device to provide quantitative information of ONH structures.[22] These include

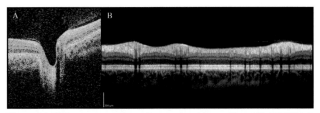

Figure 5-3. (A) B-scan across the optic nerve head from a Cirrus HD-OCT (Zeiss). (B) A circular B-scan around the optic nerve head from Spectralis OCT (Heidelberg Engineering). The retinal layers can be clearly identified.

parameters such as rim area, cup-to-disc ratio, RNFL thickness, and more. cSLO parameters have been shown to provide good discrimination between healthy and glaucomatous eyes.[22,24]

The introduction of optical coherence technology (OCT) in 1991 had an important impact on ONH imaging. OCT uses the principle of low coherence interferometry[25] to obtain high-quality images of the ONH and retinal layers. In the context of glaucoma, OCT accurately measures RNFL and macular thickness, as well as ONH parameters, such as cup-to-disc ratio, rim area, cup volume, and rim volume. The reproducibility and high diagnostic sensitivity and specificity of OCT images have made this technology the cornerstone of ONH imaging.[26]

In OCT, light emanating from a light source is split into a reference beam and a sample beam. The reference beam is directed onto a mirror and the sample beam is directed into the retina.[27] The light reflected from the 2 paths forms an interference pattern that allows the OCT machine to detect retinal layers. Multiple depthwise scans through the retina (A-scans) are combined laterally to produce a cross-sectional view of the retina (B-scan). The B-scan clearly delineates the various retinal layers (Figure 5-3).

OCT technology has evolved significantly since its introduction, particularly with regard to detection techniques.[28] The first OCT devices were known as time domain OCT (TD-OCT). In TD-OCT, the reference mirror is mechanically translated along the propagation direction of light.[29] The reference beam generates interference patterns with light reflecting from corresponding depths within the retina.[29] TD-OCT devices can acquire around 400 A-scans per second, a rate limited by the physical movement of the reference mirror. They produce images with a resolution of 10 to 15 µm.[30]

Spectral domain OCT (SD-OCT) was introduced in 2006, with the main difference from TD-OCT being the use of a stationary reference mirror. Instead of using a single point detector, like TD-OCT, in SD-OCT the returning light beams are spread using a diffraction grating and the spectrum is captured by a camera.[29] A Fourier transform is applied to the spectrum to acquire the reflectivity as a function of depth.[29] Because it is freed from the limitation of a moving mirror, SD-OCT can acquire 20,000 to 100,000 A-scans per second. It produces images with an axial resolution approaching 3 µm.[30] The transverse resolution of OCT depends on the minimal distance between adjacent sampling points and the optical properties of the eye, limiting it to the range of 15 to 20 µm. The vastly improved scan speed and number of sampling points decreases the impact of motion artifacts and improves the likelihood of picking up structural damage.[30]

RNFL thickness and ONH parameters are automatically determined by the OCT software without the need for manual delineation (Figure 5-4).[31] These parameters are reproducible with high diagnostic capability in distinguishing healthy and glaucomatous eyes, although this varies based on the severity of disease.[26] Various algorithms for automated segmentation have been described in the literature.[32-34] Most approaches use a preprocessing step to improve the OCT image quality, followed by interface detection and postprocessing.[35] The algorithm then automatically calculates the thickness of the individual retinal layers.[32] New advances in this field include using deep learning to de-noise images in the preprocessing step.[36]

The most commonly used OCT ONH parameter for glaucoma diagnosis and monitoring is the circumpapillary RNFL thickness. This sampling pattern captures the retinal ganglion cell axons from the entire retina as they approach the ONH, offering the advantage of sampling the entire retina in one pass. The global or sectoral RNFL thickness has been shown to provide superb glaucoma diagnostic and monitoring by many publications.[37-40] Other ONH parameters of importance for diagnosis and monitoring include the cup-to-disc ratio, cup area, and minimal rim width.[3,13,41,42]

NEW FRONTIERS IN IMAGING

Studies have shown that peripapillary vessel densities in glaucomatous eyes are significantly lower than in healthy eyes.[7,43] OCT angiography (OCTA) is a recently introduced iteration of OCT that allows for detailed mapping of ocular vasculature. The device acquires multiple OCT images in a short sequence and identifies locations with pixel movement between images. Because solid tissue is not expected to move in a short period of time, the moving pixels are considered to be the blood flowing through the blood vessels, which enables their mapping (Figure 5-5). When compared to conventional structural markers, quantitative measures of peripapillary vessel density have been shown to perform similarly to RNFL thickness in differentiating between healthy and glaucomatous eyes.[6] Furthermore, the association between vessel density and visual field losses are stronger than the association between RNFL thickness or rim area and visual field losses.[43] Vessel density as measured by OCTA is significantly lower in eyes with early-stage glaucoma compared to normal eyes.[44]

Another biomarker that is of interest with ocular imaging is the lamina cribrosa. Over the course of glaucomatous disease, this region of the eye undergoes a number of changes as part of the ONH remodeling process.[45] In a study of early experimental glaucoma in nonhuman primates, an increased anterior lamina cribrosa surface depth and decreased minimum rim width thickness was noted when compared to healthy eyes.[46] In glaucomatous human eyes, physical defects in the lamina, such as laminar holes and laminar disinsertions, were reported to be spatially associated with neuroretinal rim loss.[47] Others reported significant differences between healthy and glaucomatous eyes in the 3-dimensional lamina structure with parameters such as the ratio

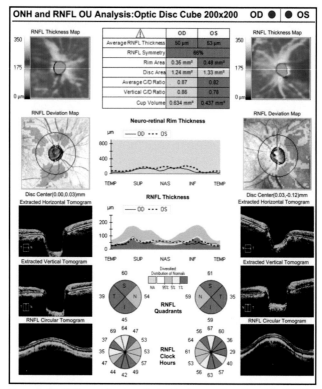

Figure 5-4A. OCT report from a patient with glaucoma from Cirrus HD-OCT. The report contains measurements of overall and sectorial RNFL thickness, and the ONH with color-coded comparison with normative data (center column). RNFL thickness map and deviation from normal maps are provided in the sides to facilitate detection of RNFL thinning marked by red and yellow regions.

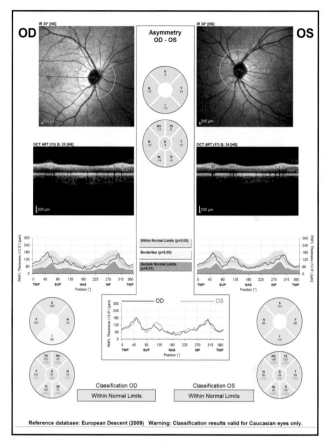

Figure 5-4B. OCT scan report of a healthy individual on a Spectralis OCT. Scan location is marked on the top fundus image with a corresponding cross section image and RNFL thickness profile underneath. Global and sectoral RNFL thickness are reported at the bottom with color-coded comparisons with normative data.

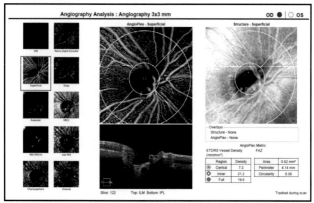

Figure 5-5A. 3 x 3 mm ONH OCTA scan report of a healthy patient from a Cirrus HD-OCT Angioplex (Zeiss). The report contains images of the peripapillary vasculature at different scan depths (left column and top right). Sectoral vessel density are measurements provided in the lower right corner.

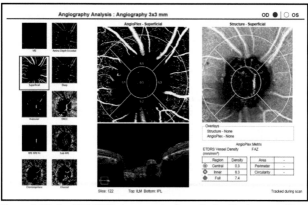

Figure 5-5B. An ONH OCTA scan report of a patient with glaucoma (Cirrus HD-OCT Angioplex) showing marked attenuation of the microvascular network.

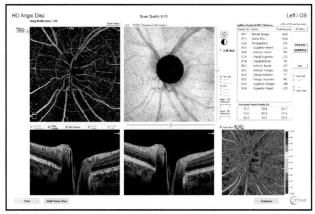

Figure 5-5C. 4.5 x 4.5 mm ONH OCTA scan report of a healthy patient from an Angiovue (Optovue) device. This device also provides quantitative vessel density information (top right) along with a color-coded vessel density map (bottom right).

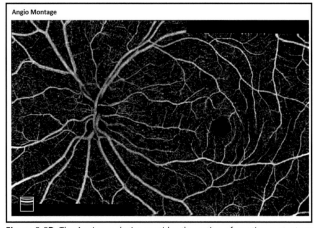

Figure 5-5D. The Angiovue device provides the option of creating a montage image, in which 6 x 6 mm OCTA images of the ONH and macula are stitched together to form an overall picture of the retinal vasculature.

between beam thickness and pore thickness.[45] Glaucomatous eyes also have a significantly more tortuous pore path within the lamina in comparison with healthy eyes, exposing the axons passing through them to axonal flow impairment.[48] While it is unclear if this is the cause for the glaucoma damage or the outcome of the remodeling process of the ONH, these findings indicate that further studies are needed to determine the role of the lamina cribrosa glaucoma.

An approach for enhancing ocular imaging quality is the incorporation of adaptive optics (AO). AO use adaptive, corrective optical elements to compensate for optical aberrations.[49] A waveform sensor measures the characteristics of optic aberrations within the eye, and the adaptive element, usually a deformable mirror, changes shape to correct for the aberrations.[49] Use of AO technology mounted on cSLO or OCT allows for improved visualization of RPE cells, leukocytes in the retinal vasculature, and individual rod and cone photoreceptor cells.[49] AO may open exciting new horizons in glaucoma imaging and improve our understanding of the pathogenesis of the disease.

A major limitation of ocular imaging quantification is the wide variation in ocular structure in healthy eyes. Even a measurement within the normal range might actually represent a substantial loss if that eye initially had thicker than normal structures. Another potential clinical scenario is a thinner than usual ocular structure that remains stable over time. This inevitable shortfall of all methods for quantifying ocular structures can be mitigated by following subjects over time while tracing structural changes. Changes that exceed changes expected in the general population likely represent abnormal findings and in the context of glaucoma represent glaucomatous damage. Many of the commercially available OCT devices provide outputs in their operating software that mark longitudinal changes and thus facilitate detection of glaucomatous damage.

Imaging of the ONH is a central component in the evaluation and management of glaucoma. It provides invaluable insights into the severity of the disease and can be used for sensitive monitoring of disease progression. Improving the ability to diagnose and track changes will allow clinicians to modulate treatment more efficiently to halt any further worsening of the disease. Eventually, as our understanding of the structural elements of glaucoma improves, new targets for the treatment of this insidious disease may emerge.

REFERENCES

1. Michelessi M, Lucenteforte E, Oddone F, et al. Optic nerve head and fibre layer imaging for diagnosing glaucoma. *The Cochrane Database Syst Rev.* 2015;11:CD008803.

2. Sommer A, Katz J, Quigley HA, et al. Clinically detectable nerve fiber atrophy precedes the onset of glaucomatous field loss. *Arch Ophthalmol.* 1991;109:77-83.

3. Pederson JE, Anderson DR. The mode of progressive disc cupping in ocular hypertension and glaucoma. *Arch Ophthalmol.* 1980;98:490-495.

4. Kerrigan-Baumrind LA, Quigley HA, Pease ME, Kerrigan DF, Mitchell RS. Number of ganglion cells in glaucoma eyes compared with threshold visual field tests in the same persons. *Invest Ophthalmol Vis Sci.* 2000;41:741-748.

5. Puchalla JL, Schneidman E, Harris RA, Berry MJ. Redundancy in the population code of the retina. *Neuron.* 2005;46:493-504.

6. Jia Y, Morrison JC, Tokayer J, et al. Quantitative OCT angiography of optic nerve head blood flow. *Biomed Opt Express.* 2012;3:3127-3137.

7. Yarmohammadi A, Zangwill LM, Diniz-Filho A, et al. Optical coherence tomography angiography vessel density in healthy, glaucoma suspect, and glaucoma eyes. *Invest Ophthalmol Vis Sci.* 2016;57:OCT451-459.

8. Wollstein G, Garway-Heath DF, Hitchings RA. Identification of early glaucoma cases with the scanning laser ophthalmoscope. *Ophthalmology.* 1998;105:1557-1563.

9. Reus NJ, Lemij HG, Garway-Heath DF, et al. Clinical assessment of stereoscopic optic disc photographs for glaucoma: the European Optic Disc Assessment Trial. *Ophthalmology.* 2010;117:717-723.

10. Schuman JS, Hee MR, Puliafito CA, et al. Quantification of nerve fiber layer thickness in normal and glaucomatous eyes using optical coherence tomography: a pilot study. *Arch Ophthalmol.* 1995;113:586-596.

11. Lavinsky F, Wu M, Schuman JS, et al. Can macula and optic nerve head parameters detect glaucoma progression in eyes with advanced circumpapillary retinal nerve fiber layer damage? *Ophthalmology.* 2018;125:1907-1912.

12. McKinnon SJ. The value of stereoscopic optic disc photography. *J Glaucoma.* 2005;3:31-33.

13. Hoffmann EM, Zangwill LM, Crowston JG, Weinreb RN. Optic disc size and glaucoma. *Surv Ophthalmol.* 2007;52:32-49.

14. Heijl A, Bengtsson B. Diagnosis of early glaucoma with flicker comparisons of serial disc photographs. *Invest Ophthalmol Vis Sci.* 1989;30:2376-2384.

15. Van Tassel SH. Optic disc hemorrhage. Edited by Sarwat Salim, EyeWiki, American Academy of Ophthalmology. eyewiki.aao.org/ Optic_Disc_Hemorrhage.

16. Law SK., Choe R, Caprioli J. Optic disk characteristics before the occurrence of disk hemorrhage in glaucoma patients. *Am J Ophthalmol.* 2001;132:411-413.

17. Prata TS, De Moraes CGV, Teng CC, et al. Factors affecting rates of visual field progression in glaucoma patients with optic disc hemorrhage. *Ophthalmology.* 2010;117:24-29.

18. Kitazawa Y, Shirato S, Yamamoto T. Optic disc hemorrhage in low-tension glaucoma. *Ophthalmology.* 1986;93:853-857.

19. Manjunath V, Shah H, Fujimoto JG, Duker JS. Analysis of peripapillary atrophy using spectral domain optical coherence tomography. *Ophthalmology.* 2011;118:531-536.

20. Park KH, Tomita G, Liou SY, Kitazawa Y. Correlation between peripapillary atrophy and optic nerve damage in normal-tension glaucoma. *Ophthalmology.* 1996;103:1899-1906.

21. Dai Y, Jonas JB, Huang H, Wang M, Sun X. Microstructure of parapapillary atrophy: beta zone and gamma zone. *Invest Ophthalmol Vis Sci.* 2013;54:2013-2018.

22. Burgansky-Eliash Z, Wollstein G, Bilonick RA, et al. Glaucoma detection with the Heidelberg retina tomograph 3. *Ophthalmology.* 2007;114:466-471.

23. Podoleanu AG, Rosen RB. Combinations of techniques in imaging the retina with high resolution. *Prog Retin Eye Res.* 2008;27:464-499.

24. Wollstein G, Garway-Heath DF, Hitchings RA. Identification of early glaucoma cases with the scanning laser ophthalmoscope. *Ophthalmology.* 1998;105:1557-1563.

25. Huang D, Swanson EA, Lin CP, et al. Optical coherence tomography. *Science.* 1991;254:1178-1181.

26. Bussel II, Wollstein G, Schuman JS. OCT for glaucoma diagnosis, screening and detection of glaucoma progression. *Br J Ophthalmol.* 2014;98(Suppl 2):ii15-ii19.

27. Schmitt JM. Optical coherence tomography (OCT): a review. *IEEE J Sel Top Quantum Electron.* 1999;5:1205-1215.

28. Gabriele ML, Wollstein G, Ishikawa H, et al. Optical coherence tomography: history, current status, and laboratory work. *Invest Ophthalmol Vis Sci.* 2011;52:2425-2436.

29. Popescu DP, Choo-Smith LP, Flueraru C, et al. Optical coherence tomography: fundamental principles, instrumental designs and biomedical applications. *Biophys Rev.* 2011;3:155-169.

30. Spirn MJ. Optical coherence tomography. EyeWiki. American Academy of Ophthalmology. eyewiki.aao.org/Optical_Coherence_ Tomography#Time_Domain_vs._Spectral_Domain.5B2.5D.

31. Lai E, Wollstein G, Price LL, et al. Optical coherence tomography disc assessment in optic nerves with peripapillary atrophy. *Ophthalmic Surg Lasers Imaging.* 2003;34:498-504.

32. Ishikawa H, Stein DM, Wollstein G, et al. Macular segmentation with optical coherence tomography. *Invest Ophthalmol Vis Sci.* 2005;46:2012-2017.

33. Koozekanani D, Boyer K, Roberts C. Retinal thickness measurements from optical coherence tomography using a Markov boundary model. *IEEE Trans Med Imaging.* 2001;20:900-916.

34. Baroni M, Fortunato P, La Torre A. Towards quantitative analysis of retinal features in optical coherence tomography. *Med Eng Phys.* 2007;29:432-441.

35. Ghorbel I, Rossant F, Bloch I, Tick S, Paques M. Automated segmentation of macular layers in OCT images and quantitative evaluation of performances. *Pattern Recognit.* 2011;44:1590-1603.

36. Halupka KJ, Antony BJ, Lee MH, et al. Retinal optical coherence tomography image enhancement via deep learning. *Biomed Opt Express.* 2018;9:6205-6221.

37. Medeiros FA, Zangwill LM, Bowd C, et al. Evaluation of retinal nerve fiber layer, optic nerve head, and macular thickness measurements for glaucoma detection using optical coherence tomography. *Am J Ophthalmol.* 2005;139:44-55.

38. Kanamori A, Nakamura M, Escano MFT, et al. Evaluation of the glaucomatous damage on retinal nerve fiber layer thickness measured by optical coherence tomography. *Am J Ophthalmol.* 2003;135:513-520.

39. Bowd C, Weinreb RN, Williams JM, Zangwill LM. The retinal nerve fiber layer thickness in ocular hypertensive, normal, and glaucomatous eyes with optical coherence tomography. *Arch Ophthalmol.* 2000;118:22-26.

40. Wollstein G, Schuman JS, Price LL, et al.. Optical coherence tomography longitudinal evaluation of retinal nerve fiber layer thickness in glaucoma. *Arch Ophthalmol.* 2005;123:464-470.

41. Airaksinen PJ, Tuulonen A, Alanko HI. Rate and pattern of neuroretinal rim area decrease in ocular hypertension and glaucoma. *Arch Ophthalmol.* 1992;110:206-210.

42. Jonas JB, Budde WM, Lang P. Neuroretinal rim width ratios in morphological glaucoma diagnosis. *Br J Ophthalmol.* 1998;82:1366-1371.

43. Yarmohammadi A, Zangwill LM, Diniz-Filho A, et al. Relationship between optical coherence tomography angiography vessel density and severity of visual field loss in glaucoma. *Ophthalmology.* 2016;123:2498-2508.

44. Hou H, Moghimi S, Zangwill LM, et al. Macula vessel density and thickness in early primary open-angle glaucoma. *Am J Ophthalmol.* 2019;199:120-132.

45. Wang B, Nevins JE, Nadler Z, et al. In vivo lamina cribrosa micro-architecture in healthy and glaucomatous eyes as assessed by optical coherence tomography. *Invest Ophthalmol Vis Sci.* 2013;54:8270-8274.

46. Ivers KM, Sredar N, Patel NB, et al. In vivo changes in lamina cribrosa microarchitecture and optic nerve head structure in early experimental glaucoma. *PloS One*. 2015;10:e0134223.

47. You JY, Park SC, Su D, et al. Focal lamina cribrosa defects associated with glaucomatous rim thinning and acquired pits. *JAMA Ophthalmol*. 2013;131:314-320.

48. Wang B, Lucy KA, Schuman JS, et al. Tortuous pore path through the glaucomatous lamina cribrosa. *Scientific Reports*. 2018;8:7281.

49. Godara P, Dubis AM, Roorda A, Duncan JL, Carroll J. Adaptive optics retinal imaging: emerging clinical applications. *Optom Vis Sci*. 2010;87:930-941.

6

Visual Fields
What I Need to Know

*Ahmad A. Aref, MD, MBA
and Donald L. Budenz, MD, MPH*

ROLE OF PERIMETRY IN
GLAUCOMA MANAGEMENT

Progressive glaucomatous optic neuropathy may be characterized by structural alterations in the optic disc, peripapillary retinal nerve fiber layer, and macula, that often precede corresponding detectable changes in visual function. The two parameters—
structure and function—are both essential and complimentary
in the assessment and monitoring of glaucomatous individuals
to allow for timely treatment and visual preservation. Standard
automated perimetry (SAP) remains a universally accepted and
widely utilized method for the assessment of visual function in
the setting of glaucomatous disease. This chapter will discuss
various SAP testing protocols in addition to pearls and pitfalls in
interpretation of the standard results printout. Current methods
for glaucoma staging and detection of progression will also be
discussed.

Panarelli JF, ed.
The Pocket Guide to Glaucoma (pp 73-90).
© 2022 Taylor & Francis Group.

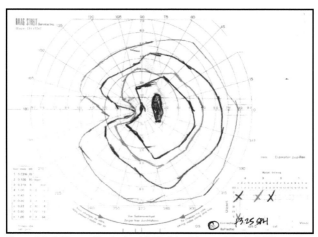

Figure 6-1. Goldmann kinetic visual field of the right eye. Stimuli of different sizes are moved from the periphery toward fixation until a patient response is elicited. Isopters corresponding to the respective stimuli are color coded to generate a map of the entire visual field. This patient suffers superior and inferior nasal steps that become gradually more exaggerated as stimulus size decreases.

KINETIC VERSUS AUTOMATED STATIC PERIMETRY

Kinetic perimetric techniques involve the use of visual targets, each of specified size and luminance, that are moved from a patient's peripheral field toward the center, with color coded recording of the first detection in various regions that are connected to form isopters and a sensitivity map (Figure 6-1). Goldmann kinetic perimetry allows for measurement of sensitivity across the entire visual field and is therefore useful for determining overall visual function and ability to perform specified activities, such as driving. However, kinetic perimetry is highly technician-dependent and time-intensive.

Automated, static techniques involve the use of stationary stimuli of a given size that vary in luminance. The luminance threshold in a given testing location for an individual patient is determined by presenting a wide range of attenuated light stimuli within the testing range and then determining the dimmest sensitivity seen 50% of the time.

Given the relative subjectivity of kinetic perimetry and the quantitative nature of automated techniques, static perimetry is most often preferred for the diagnosis and follow-up of glaucomatous patients.

AUTOMATED VISUAL FIELD TESTING PROTOCOLS

Field Range

The most commonly employed testing range for the purposes of glaucoma management is the central 24-degree field in addition to 2 nasal points measured out to 30 degrees. This 24-2 protocol consists of 54 testing points spaced 6 degrees apart. A 30-degree field (protocol 30-2) may be used also, but edge points within this protocol are subject to high degrees of variability and error and are typically ignored. A central 10-degree field (protocol 10-2) has utility in advanced disease states, and growing evidence now suggests a role in milder disease as well.[1]

Stimulus Size

Visual field testing stimulus sizes range from Goldmann size 0 (1/16 mm^2) to Goldmann size V (64 mm^2). For the majority of patients, a size III stimulus (4 mm^2) is chosen, and this is the standard in the 24-2 testing protocol. For patients with Snellen visual acuity less than 20/80, a size V stimulus may be more appropriate.

Testing Strategy

Swedish Interactive Testing Algorithm Standard

The Swedish Interactive Testing Algorithm (SITA) uses Bayesian probability techniques to estimate locational threshold sensitivities with greatest accuracy while reducing testing time.[2] The SITA Standard testing algorithm estimates the likelihood of threshold sensitivity based on patient age, testing location, and previous responses. This strategy is employed, rather than testing every single stimulus strength at every location. In that way, SITA Standard testing can be reduced to an average of 7 minutes per eye.

Swedish Interactive Testing Algorithm Fast

The SITA Fast protocol uses larger steps when presenting stimuli in various locations within the visual field. By presenting a lower number of stimuli intensities, the test may save time compared to SITA Standard techniques. However, this benefit often trades off testing accuracy with an increase in measurement variability and error, most pronounced in testing locations of lower sensitivity.[3] In addition, SITA Fast may have lower sensitivity for glaucomatous defect detection.[4]

Swedish Interactive Testing Algorithm Faster

A novel technique designed to replace SITA Fast testing protocols was recently described by Heijl et al.[5] The SITA Faster technique modifies the SITA Fast strategy in 7 ways to allow for more rapid testing time without compromising test-retest variability. Notably, the SITA Faster technique starts testing with luminance age-matched average attenuation levels, rather than supraliminal levels of 25 db. The SITA Faster technique also does not retest areas where the patient has previously not responded to a stimulus intensity of 0 dB.

Swedish Interactive Testing Algorithm Short-Wavelength Automated Perimetery

Short-Wavelength Automated Perimetery (SWAP) is intended to test sensitivity of the blue-yellow ganglion cells, which are believed to be more sensitive than the remaining ganglion cell population to glaucomatous damage. To specifically target this population, a yellow background is used to adapt rods and cones that send signals to non–blue-yellow ganglion cells. A blue, size V stimulus is then used to target short-wavelength sensitive cones that send signals to blue-yellow ganglion cells. In comparison to standard perimetric techniques, SWAP has been shown to detect glaucomatous onset and progression at earlier time points. One disadvantage of SWAP testing techniques is that lenticular opacities and age-related macular degeneration, both common in the older patient with glaucoma, may attenuate the stimulus signal and lead to decreased diagnostic accuracy.[6]

Full Threshold

Full threshold testing involves a "staircase" testing algorithm that initially tests each location with successively attenuated stimuli in 4 dB steps. After an instance of no response, successively less attenuated stimuli are administered in 2 dB steps until a positive response is elicited. Full threshold strategies do not use Bayesian probability techniques to predict response and, therefore, present each location with a greater number of stimuli, resulting in longer testing time. Due to differences in measurement of global indices and focal defect depth, practitioners should not compare full threshold to SITA Standard test results when assessing glaucomatous loss.[7]

Suprathreshold

Rather than grading the attenuation of a signal in order to quantify sensitivity, suprathreshold techniques use stimuli that are likely to be more luminous than a patient's threshold sensitivity based on age and testing location. The test then assesses whether or not the patient responds to the stimulus in a given location. Suprathreshold testing is mostly used to evaluate visual field disability, often with criteria for specific functions, such as driving or prior to ptosis surgery.

INTERPRETING THE SWEDISH INTERACTIVE TESTING ALGORITHM STANDARD 24-2, SIZE III SINGLE FIELD ANALYSIS PRINTOUT

Visual Field Test Type

The top of the test results printout (Figure 6-2) indicates important information regarding testing parameters, such as field range, testing strategy, test stimulus size, and background illumination levels.[8] It is important to confirm that this information corresponds to desired testing methods under the clinical circumstances.

Patient Demographics and Clinical Characteristics

Patient characteristics and demographics are listed at the top of the printout. These include patient name, age, birth date, date of visual field test, patient identification number, physiologic pupil diameter, visual acuity, and correction used to administer the test. It is critical for the clinician to confirm the accuracy of this information prior to proceeding with field interpretation and clinical decision making.

Reliability Indices

Fixation Loss Rate

The patient's fixation is tested by presenting a number of stimuli in the perimetric blind spot, once this has been mapped. Responses to these stimuli are presumed to be secondary to deviation of patient fixation from the central target. The ratio of fixation loss to total presentations is then given in the printout

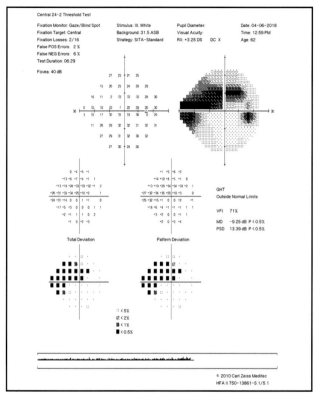

Figure 6-2. Standard 24-2, SITA Standard automated visual field test printout. Reliability indices are shown in the top left-hand side of the printout. Foveal threshold is noted just below the reliability indices. In this example depicting advanced glaucomatous loss, the foveal threshold is within normal range. The top middle section of the printout indicates the stimulus size, background illumination level, and testing strategy. The middle of the printout displays raw threshold sensitivities in decibels adjacent to a graytone image depicting the general pattern of loss. Below these maps are the total and pattern deviation plots, which show deviation of each point's sensitivity from age-matched controls both numerically and with gray-scaled boxes according to percentile rank. On the right-hand side of the printout just under the graytone map, are the global indices that show results of the Glaucoma Hemifield Test, as well as the visual field index, mean deviation, and pattern standard deviation. The gaze tracker at the bottom of the printout gives a sense of how well the patient fixated throughout the test, with upward deflections indicating gaze deviation from fixation.

with an "XX" placed next to the ratio once the percentage of loss exceeds 20%. Incorrect blind spot mapping and/or a generally high false positive rate may also lead to presumption of fixation loss. High fixation loss rates may underestimate visual field loss in glaucomatous individuals.

False Positive Errors

The testing machine will occasionally produce mechanical noises and time delay in absence of presentation of the visual stimulus. If a patient responds to this series of events, a false positive error is recorded. The ratio of false positive responses to presentations is given in the printout with an "XX" placed next to the ratio once the percentage of loss exceeds 20%. As with the fixation loss rate, it is important to note the false positive rate, as it may lead to underestimation of visual field loss.

False Negative Errors

If a patient fails to respond to stimulation that is brighter than the previously determined sensitivity threshold for a given location, a false negative error is recorded. High false negative rates lead to unreliable visual fields, usually indicate patient inattentiveness and fatigue, and lead to overestimation of visual field loss.

Is the Field Test Abnormal?

Threshold Printout

The threshold printout provides numerical average sensitivity values for each tested location in units of decibels, corresponding to attenuation of light. Higher decibel values correspond to dimmer stimuli.

Foveal Threshold

The beginning of the test involves presentation of a stimulus just inferior to the central fixation light within the perimetry bowl. This is used to determine the foveal threshold value, which is displayed in the top left corner of the results printout. If the foveal threshold differs from age-matched controls, an accompanying *P*-value is given. A significantly abnormal foveal threshold often indicates ocular pathology independent from the glaucomatous disease process.

Graytone Printout

The graytone map is displayed in the top right corner of the results printout. The map provides a gross graphical representation of the degree of field abnormality and also the pattern of loss.

Total Deviation Printout and Probability Plot

The total deviation plot displays the numerical deviation of sensitivity values from age-matched controls in each testing location. The accompanying total deviation probability plot assigns a gray-scaled box to each location based on age-matched percentile rank (top 95% [no shading], lower 5%, lower 2%, lower 1%, and lower .5% [black shading]).

Pattern Deviation Printout and Probability Plot

The average amount of loss in the threshold deviation plot is determined and then used to generate the pattern deviation plot, which removes the effect of diffuse depression. This method allows for isolation of focal defects more likely to be neurologic/glaucomatous rather than ocular surface or lenticular in nature. A pattern probability plot is generated with corresponding gray-scale-toned boxes as indicated for the threshold probability plot.

Global Indices

Mean Deviation

The average of individual deviations in threshold sensitivity values from age-matched controls gives the mean deviation value, which is indicated in the lower-right of the printout. An accompanying *P*-value is given to indicate percentile rank.

Visual Field Index

The visual field index (VFI) provides a measure of percentage of remaining perimetric vision and is closely related to the mean deviation. Importantly, it is calculated from the pattern deviation sensitivity plot and is therefore adjusted for areas of diffuse depression that are likely nonglaucomatous. The VFI also weighs central points more than peripheral ones. To calculate the VFI, areas of normal sensitivity on the pattern deviation plot are considered to be 100%, even if depression is noted on the total deviation plot.

Pattern Standard Deviation

Just under the mean deviation is the pattern standard deviation, which is a measure of the degree of localized depression, adjusting for diffuse loss. An accompanying P-value is given to indicate percentile rank. An abnormal pattern standard deviation can be an early indicator of localized defects from glaucoma and other disorders that cause localized loss of the visual field.

Glaucoma Hemifield Test

The threshold sensitivity of 5 clusters of points (corresponding anatomically to nerve fiber layer segments) in the superior and inferior hemifields are compared in the Glaucoma Hemifield Test (GHT). The GHT may be classified as "within normal limits," "borderline," "outside normal limits," "general reduction in sensitivity," or "abnormally high sensitivity" based on the degree of asymmetry compared to age-matched controls. Results of the GHT have been found to have high levels of diagnostic accuracy for determining the presence or absence of glaucomatous optic neuropathy. However, it is important to note that not all abnormalities of GHT are due to glaucoma.

SEVERITY STAGING

Hodapp-Anderson-Parrish Criteria

The Hodapp-Anderson-Parrish Criteria (Table 6-1) for glaucoma staging on the basis of SAP were developed in 1993.[9] The criteria are useful for making an early diagnosis of glaucoma and also for grading severity in order to guide treatment goals. The criteria take into account generalized and focal loss, as well as location with respect to fixation.

ICD-10 Staging Criteria

The International Statistical Classification of Diseases and Related Health Problems (ICD) is a coding system maintained by the World Health Organization for global health statistics and medical billing. The 10th version of this coding system (ICD-10) allows for the practitioner to classify glaucoma severity on the basis of stage (Table 6-2), with criteria dependent on visual field characteristics.

ASSESSING PROGRESSION

Although subjective judgment based on review of serial visual field tests may be used to assess for functional glaucomatous progression, these methods are subjective and nonstandardized compared to event- and trend-based analyses (Figure 6-3) generated using perimetric statistical software.[10]

Event-Based Analysis

Event-based analyses determine glaucomatous progression on the basis of worsening focal defects over time. The Guided Progression Analysis (GPA; Zeiss) compares the threshold sensitivity of each point on the pattern deviation plot with the average sensitivity of the same point on 2 baseline tests. When 3 testing

Table 6-1. Hodapp-Anderson-Parrish Glaucoma Staging Criteria

MINIMAL GLAUCOMATOUS ABNORMALITY
(ONE OF THE FOLLOWING, MUST BE REPRODUCIBLE)

Three or more adjacent, nonedge points in a location of the central 24-degree field typical for glaucoma, all of which are depressed to a *P*-value less than 5% on the pattern deviation plot and 1 of which is depressed to *P* < 1%

A GHT outside normal limits

A corrected pattern standard deviation with *P*-value < 5%

A diffusely depressed total deviation plot with mean deviation depressed at a *P*-value < 5% with no other nonglaucomatous explanation for depression and with corresponding clinical findings consistent with glaucoma

EARLY GLAUCOMATOUS DEFECT
(ALL OF THE FOLLOWING)

Mean deviation better than -6 dB

All points in the central 5 degrees with sensitivity ≥ 15 dB

Less than 25% of the points (18) are depressed to *P* < 5% and less than 10 points are depressed to *P* < 1% on the pattern deviation plot

MODERATE GLAUCOMATOUS DEFECT
(ALL OF THE FOLLOWING)

Mean deviation better than -12 dB

Less than 50% of the points (37) are depressed to *P* < 5% and less than 20 points are depressed to *P* < 1% on the pattern deviation plot

Only one hemifield may have a point with sensitivity < 15 dB and within 5 degrees of fixation

(continued)

Table 6-1. Hodapp-Anderson-Parrish Glaucoma Staging Criteria (continued)

SEVERE GLAUCOMATOUS DEFECT
(ALL OF THE FOLLOWING)

Mean deviation worse than -12 dB

More than 50% of the points (37) are depressed to $P < 5\%$ or more than 20 points are depressed to $P < 1\%$ on the pattern deviation plot

Points within the central 5 degrees with sensitivity < 15 dB in both hemifields

GHT = Glaucoma Hemifield Test.

Adapted from Anderson RD, Patella VM. *Automated Static Perimetry*, 2nd ed. Mosby; 1999

Table 6-2. ICD-10 Glaucoma Staging Criteria

MILD-/EARLY-STAGE GLAUCOMA

No visual field defect consistent with glaucoma in the presence of structural glaucomatous abnormalities

MODERATE-STAGE GLAUCOMA
(ALL OF THE FOLLOWING)

Glaucomatous defect in only 1 hemifield

No glaucomatous defect within 5 degrees of fixation

SEVERE-STAGE GLAUCOMA
(ONE OF THE FOLLOWING)

Glaucomatous defect in both hemifields

Glaucomatous defect within 5 degrees of fixation in at least 1 hemifield

INDETERMINATE-STAGE GLAUCOMA

Visual fields not performed

Patient incapable of visual field testing

Unreliable/uninterpretable visual field testing

Reproduced from the Centers for Medicare & Medicaid Services.

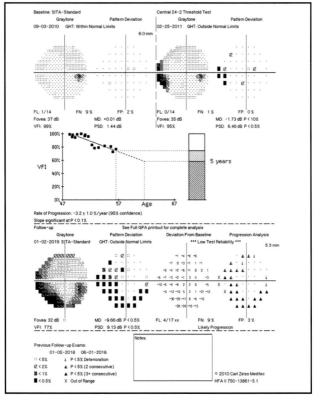

Figure 6-3. Automated visual field results showing glaucomatous progression, as shown by both trend-based and event-based methodologies and the GPA. The regression line in the middle of the printout predicts ongoing perimetric loss over the next 5 years. Completely shaded triangles in the lower right plot correspond to locations of progressively depressed points confirmed on 2 examinations subsequent to baseline studies.

points in the follow-up study exceed deterioration outside of the 95% confidence interval of test-retest variability in a group of stable glaucoma patients with confirmation on 1 subsequent test, a determination of "possible progression" is indicated. If worsening is reproduced and confirmed on 3 consecutive tests at the exact 3 locations, "likely progression" is indicated. Once the clinician has made a determination of progression and managed accordingly, it is important to re-establish a new benchmark by exchanging the 2 initial baseline studies with the more recent tests. Otherwise, the "likely progression" message will persist despite stabilization of the visual field.

Trend-Based Analysis

Trend-based analyses use global measures to determine overall functional progression. The GPA uses regression analysis of the VFI parameter over time to determine the rate of perimetric loss. Computerized extrapolation of the VFI trend then predicts the percentage of expected perimetric loss over the next 5 years. Trend-based techniques are often more useful in moderate and severe stages of glaucomatous disease, whereas event-based analysis may be more sensitive in mild stages.

PITFALLS AND ARTIFACTS

Role of the Perimetrist

Although SAP is considered a quantitative test, several qualitative variables may impact testing results and accuracy. Patient attentiveness throughout the test will likely influence the rate of false positives, false negatives, and fixation losses. To this end, it is important for the perimetrist to explain the goals of the test, situate the patient comfortably, and stay engaged throughout the test. The perimtrist should also provide reassurance to the patient that a stimulus may not be seen for over half of the testing time and that stimuli will likely appear relatively dim when seen.[11]

Instructing the patient to press the button when they think they see a light will help with this. It may also help for the perimetrist to instruct the patient to hold the response button down if they want to pause the test to take a break or speak to the perimetrist. We do not advocate 1 perimetrist conducting 2 visual field tests at the same time or having 2 visual field tests occurring in the same room. These strategies will help patients develop a positive attitude toward perimetry over their treatment course.

Media Opacification

Diseases of the cornea, lens, and vitreous may lead to visual field loss that can confound interpretation for glaucoma diagnostic purposes. Because these disorders usually lead to diffuse rather than focal depression, it is important for the practitioner to place greater weight on the pattern, rather than the total, deviation plot. Furthermore, these disorders are more likely to lead to reduction in the foveal threshold along with decreased central visual acuity compared to glaucomatous optic neuropathy.

Lens Rim Artifact

Malposition of the corrective lens used for testing may result in an absolute scotoma with threshold sensitivities < 0 dB. Properly distanced (as close to the patient as possible without interfering with eyelashes and/or brow) and centered corrective lenses with thinner wire rims help to minimize the frequency of this artifact.

Lid/Brow Artifact

Superior ptosis and/or a prominent forehead brow may decrease threshold sensitivity superiorly and mimic a glaucomatous arcuate defect. Superior eyelid taping and proper positioning may decrease the frequency of these artifacts.

Fatigue

Inattentiveness may occur after testing of fixation and the 4 cardinal points in each quadrant of the visual field. The classic clover leaf pattern of visual field loss often results as a consequence. Another sign of patient fatigue is a high false negative rate in the setting of normal fixation loss and false positive rates.

Pupil Size

A relatively mydriatic or miotic pupil may lead to increased and decreased levels of retinal illumination, respectively, resulting in testing artifact. A practitioner should standardize their practice such that visual fields are performed under the same pupillary conditions in order to allow for meaningful interpretation over time. For patients on chronic miotic therapy, consideration may be given to pharmacologic dilation prior to testing.

CONCLUSION

Despite all of its shortcomings, the visual field test remains the most important test of visual function in glaucoma. There are powerful computational tools available to aid in interpretation of results, and practitioners should utilize all of them to maximize diagnostic capabilities of the test. Controlling testing conditions and patient cooperation are key to successful results.

REFERENCES

1. Hood DC, Raza AS, de Moraes CG, et al. Glaucomatous damage of the macula. *Prog Retin Eye Res.* 2013;32:1-21.
2. Wild JM, Pacey IE, O'Neill EC, Cunliffe IA. The SITA perimetric threshold algorithms in glaucoma. *Invest Ophthalmol Vis Sci.* 1999;40(9):1998-2009.
3. Artes PH, Iwase A, Ohno Y, et al. Properties of perimetric threshold estimates from Full Threshold, SITA Standard, and SITA Fast strategies. *Invest Ophthalmol Vis Sci.* 2002;43(8):2654-2659.

4. Budenz DL, Rhee P, Feuer WJ, et al. Sensitivity and specificity of the Swedish interactive threshold algorithm for glaucomatous visual field defects. *Ophthalmology.* 2002;109:1052-1058.

5. Heijl A, Patella VM, Chong LX, et al. A new SITA perimetric threshold testing algorithm; construction and a multi-center clinical study. *Am J Ophthalmol.* 2019;198:154-165.

6. Niforushan N, Parsamanesh M, Yu F, et al. Effect of yellow-tinted intraocular lens on standard automated perimetry and short wavelength automated perimetry in patients with glaucoma. *Middle East Afr J Ophthalmol.* 2014;21(3):216-219.

7. Budenz DL, Rhee P, Feuer WJ, et al. Comparison of glaucomatous visual field defects using standard full threshold and Swedish interactive threshold algorithms. *Arch Ophthalmol.* 2002;120(9):1136-1141.

8. Budenz DL. *Atlas of Visual Fields.* Lippencott-Raven; 1997.

9. Anderson RD, Patella VM. *Automated Static Perimetry.* 2nd ed. Mosby; 1999.

10. Aref AA, Budenz DL. Detecting visual field progression. *Ophthalmology.* 2017;124:S51-S56.

11. Heijl A, Patella VM, Bengtsson B. *Effective Perimetry.* 4th ed. Carl Zeiss Meditec, Inc, 2012.

7

Laser Procedures for Glaucoma

J. Minjy Kang, MD
and Paul A. Sidoti, MD

LASER BASICS

The term *laser* is an acronym for light amplification by stimulated emission of radiation. Several different properties and components of lasers are relevant to their application in ophthalmology. The *gain medium* of a laser is the medium it uses in the amplification of light. Examples of different gain mediums used in ophthalmologic lasers are gas (eg, argon), solid-state (eg, Nd:YAG), and semiconductor (eg, diode). The output of a laser can either be continuous or pulsed (eg, Q-switched frequency-doubled Nd:YAG or micropulse diode laser). The absorption of laser energy by a specific chromophore will depend on the wavelength of the laser. Melanin effectively absorbs visible light, which ranges from about 380 to 740 nm. When laser is absorbed by tissue it can have one of the following effects: photocoagulation (eg, argon laser), photoablation (eg, excimer laser), and photodisruption (eg, Nd:YAG laser).

Panarelli JF, ed.
The Pocket Guide to Glaucoma (pp 91-118).
© 2022 Taylor & Francis Group.

Figure 7-1. Bombe configuration of the iris in a patient with pupillary block angle closure.

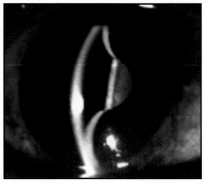

COMMON GLAUCOMA LASER PROCEDURES

Iridotomy

Laser peripheral iridotomy (LPI) is an essential tool in the management of anatomically narrow anterior chamber angles, primary angle closure (PAC), PAC glaucoma (PACG), and acute angle closure crisis (AACC). Angle closure frequently results from pupillary block, in which there is relative resistance to aqueous flow from the posterior chamber to the anterior chamber through the iridolenticular space. Pressure then builds up in the posterior chamber, causing the peripheral iris to bow forward, narrowing the space between the iris and the trabecular meshwork (Figure 7-1). Iridotrabebular contact and permanent synechial angle closure may result, preventing the outflow of aqueous through the trabecular meshwork and producing a rise in intraocular pressure (IOP). An LPI provides an alternate pathway for aqueous flow from the posterior chamber to the anterior chamber where it can access the trabecular meshwork. However, while imaging studies demonstrate an initial increase in angle width, this effect may decrease over time due to increasing lens vault.[1-3] Additionally, 19.4% to 81% of PAC suspect patients may demonstrate persistent angle closure on gonioscopy or ultrasound biomicroscopy after LPI.[4-6] Residual angle closure can occur due to nonpupillary block mechanisms, such as thicker iris, anteriorly positioned ciliary body, and greater lens vault. Therefore, it is important to continue to monitor patients with gonioscopy for angle closure even after LPI.

Indications

- Anatomically narrow anterior chamber angles
- PAC suspect
- PACG
- AACC
- Nanophthalmos
- Plateau iris configuration/syndrome
- Utility in pigmentary dispersion syndrome/glaucoma debated[7]

Contraindications

- Corneal opacification obscuring view
- Flat anterior chamber

Laser Types

- Argon, continuous wave (488, 514, 532 nm)
- Green diode, continuous wave (532 nm)
- Nd:YAG, Q switched, pulsed (1064 nm)

Laser Settings

LASER	POWER/ ENERGY	DURATION/ PULSES	SPOT SIZE
Argon/green diode (contraction/ pretreatment)	200 to 500 mW	0.2 to 0.5 sec	200 to 500 µm
Argon/green diode (penetrating)	600 to 1200 mW	0.01 to 0.05 sec	50 to 75 µm
Nd:YAG	4 to 10 mJ	1 to 3 pulses per burst	(constant; set by each laser model)

Lenses

- Abraham iridectomy
- Wise iridotomy
- Pollack iridotomy/gonio

Procedure

- Confirm correct eye to be treated and that consent has been obtained
- Instill pilocarpine 1% to 2% 15 to 30 minutes prior to procedure
  - May defer pilocarpine and utilize bright slit lamp beam to constrict pupil intraoperatively
- Pretreat with topical apraclonidine or brimonidine to minimize the risk of a postoperative IOP spike
- Instill 1 drop of proparacaine or tetracaine topical anesthetic
  - Warn patients they may feel mild discomfort from the laser applications
- Place methylcellulose or 0.3% hypromellose gel on iridotomy lens

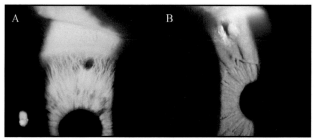

Figure 7-2. Peripheral iridotomies performed with an argon laser (A) and an Nd:YAG laser (B).

- Identify a thinner area of the peripheral iris (crypt) beyond the lens equator, avoiding blood vessels
  - Can be placed in the superior or nasal/temporal location (may be a lower incidence of postoperative dysphotopsia when placed adjacent to the horizontal meridian)[8,9]
- Apply laser (see previous Laser Settings section) until patency confirmed by visualizing flow of aqueous and pigment from the posterior to anterior chamber (Figure 7-2)
  - Consider pretreatment with continuous wave, photocoagulative laser (eg, argon or diode laser) prior to the Nd:YAG laser to thin the iris via thermal contraction and reduce the risk of bleeding
- If bleeding occurs, hold intermittent pressure on the eye using the iridotomy lens until active bleeding stops

Postoperative Care and Follow-Up

- Recheck IOP 30 to 60 minutes after procedure
- Topical steroid 3 to 4 times per day for 3 to 7 days (or longer if inflammation persists)
- Follow-up visit at 1 week to check IOP, repeat gonioscopy, and taper topical steroid, depending on the residual anterior chamber inflammatory reaction

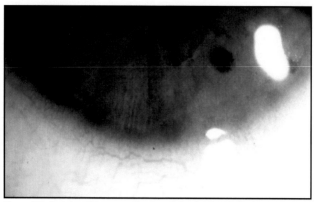

Figure 7-3. Peripheral iris contraction scars following laser iridoplasty.

Complications

- IOP spike
- Hyphema
- Inflammation
- Laser burn to cornea, lens, or retina
- Dysphotopsia
- Closure of iridotomy
- Persistent angle closure

Iridoplasty

Laser peripheral iridoplasty, or peripheral iris contraction procedure (PICP), is effective in reversing iridotrabecular apposition and opening the angle in situations where it is difficult to perform a LPI or when there is residual iridotrabecular contact in the presence of a patent LPI. When performing PICP, large-diameter, low-power (nonpenetrating) laser burns are applied to the far periphery of the iris, causing it to contract, thin, and separate from the adjacent angle structures (Figure 7-3). This has been shown to be effective in breaking AACC and can be more readily performed in cases where corneal edema or a shallow anterior chamber may preclude the successful execution of an LPI.[10,11] This procedure does not, however, eliminate pupillary block, so an LPI should be performed at a later time after the acute crisis has resolved. PICP also has a role in treating PAC(G) patients with persistent iridotrabecular apposition after LPI. It is best to document the ability to separate the iris from the trabecular meshwork with indentation gonioscopy prior to performing PICP, as this procedure will not reverse synechial angle closure. Peripheral iridoplasty alone may not be a good long-term therapeutic solution, as additional intervention or surgery is often required.[12-14]

Indications

- To open an appositionally closed angle
- AACC
- Persistent appositional angle closure in the presence of patent iridotomy without peripheral anterior synechiae
  - Plateau iris syndrome
  - Phacomorphic glaucoma (angle closure related to the size or position of the lens)
  - Nanophthalmos

Contraindications

- Severe corneal edema
- Flat anterior chamber
- Peripheral anterior synechiae

Laser Types

- Argon, continuous wave (488, 514, 532 nm)
- Red diode, continuous wave (810 nm)
- Green diode, continuous wave (532 nm)

Laser Settings

LASER	POWER	DURATION	SPOT SIZE
Argon	150 to 500 mW	0.2 to 0.5 sec	200 to 500 μm
Red diode	400 to 500 mW	0.2 to 0.3 sec	200 to 500 μm
Green diode	150 to 500 mW	0.2 to 0.5 sec	200 to 500 μm

Lenses

- Abraham iridectomy
- Wise iridotomy

In general, a gonioscopic lens is not recommended, as an angled mirror is more likely to result in inadvertent damage to the trabecular meshwork and less peripheral iris stromal contraction/thinning, due to tangential orientation of the laser.[11]

Procedure

- Confirm correct eye to be treated and that consent has been obtained
- Instill pilocarpine 1% to 2% 15 to 30 minutes prior to procedure
- Pretreat with topical apraclonidine or brimonidine to minimize the risk of a postoperative IOP spike
- Instill 1 drop of proparacaine or tetracaine topical anesthetic
  - Warn patients they may feel discomfort from the laser
- Place methylcellulose or 0.3% hypromellose gel on goniolens
- Apply laser to the far periphery of the iris (at the iris root) and titrate power to a visible endpoint of focal iris contracture without bubble formation, pigment release, or tissue penetration (see previous Laser Settings section)

- Apply 24 to 32 spots over 360 degrees, each spot about 1 to 2 spot-diameters apart
- Lighter-colored irides require more power (may be more effective with smaller spot size)

Postoperative Care and Follow-Up

- Recheck IOP 30 to 60 minutes after procedure
- Topical steroid 4 times per day for 7 days or longer as needed
- Follow-up visit to check IOP, anterior chamber inflammatory reaction, and gonioscopy

Complications

- IOP spike
- Persistent inflammation
- Corneal endothelial burns
- Transient or permanent change in pupillary shape/size

Laser Trabeculoplasty

Laser trabeculoplasty (LTP) is performed to lower IOP by applying laser energy to the trabecular meshwork with a resultant increase in aqueous outflow. Argon laser trabeculoplasty (ALT) was introduced by Wise and Witter in 1979.[15] The Glaucoma Laser Trial demonstrated the safety and efficacy of ALT as an alternative first-line treatment to topical medications for primary open-angle glaucoma (POAG).[16] Later, Latina et al described using a Q-switched, frequency-doubled Nd:YAG laser to perform selective LTP (SLT).[17] Due to the pulsed energy delivery, SLT induces less tissue damage than ALT, while maintaining a similar IOP-lowering effect.[18] The pulse duration of the laser used for SLT is shorter than the thermal relaxation time of melanin, resulting in less damage to surrounding nonpigmented cells and structures. Success rate (defined as > 20% reduction of IOP from baseline) for SLT has been reported to be 58% to 94% at 1 year,[19-23] with diminishing success over time (38% to 85% at 2 years).[19,21-23] Eyes with higher baseline IOP tend to have a greater IOP-lowering effect after SLT.[24-26] Repeat SLT (after prior ALT or SLT) appears to have similar outcomes as initial laser treatment.[27-31] Micropulse diode laser trabeculoplasty (MLT/MDLT) is a relatively newer laser procedure that, as the name suggests, also utilizes a pulsed laser and, therefore, causes less collateral tissue damage compared to continuous lasers, such as argon.[32]

Indications

- POAG
- Pigmentary glaucoma
- Pseudoexfoliative glaucoma
- Steroid-induced glaucoma

Contraindications

- Inability to visualize the trabecular meshwork
- Angle-closure glaucoma
- Neovascular glaucoma
- Inflammatory glaucoma
- Angle-recession glaucoma
- Juvenile OAG (patient age less than 40 years at diagnosis)
- Congenital glaucoma

Laser Types

- Argon (ALT); continuous wave (488, 514, 532 nm)
- Q-switched, frequency-doubled Nd:YAG (SLT); pulsed laser (532 nm)
- Red diode (MLT/MDLT); pulsed laser (810 nm)

Laser Settings

LASER	POWER/ ENERGY	DURATION	SPOT SIZE
Argon	400 to 1000 mW	0.1 sec	50 μm
Green diode	400 to 1000 mW	0.1 sec	50 to 75 μm
Q-switched, freqency-doubled Nd:YAG	0.4 to 1.2 mJ	3 ns	400 μm
Micropulse diode	1000 to 2000 mW	0.2 to 0.3 sec (15% duty cycle)	300 μm

Lenses

- Ritch trabeculoplasty
- Latina
- Goldmann 3-mirror

Procedure

- Confirm correct eye to be treated and that consent has been obtained
- Pretreat with topical apraclonidine or brimonidine to minimize the risk of a postoperative IOP spike
- Instill 1 drop of proparacaine or tetracaine topical anesthetic
- Place methylcellulose or 0.3% hypromellose gel on goniolens
- Place goniolens on eye and apply laser to pigmented trabecular meshwork (see previous Laser Settings section) for 180 to 360 degrees, 20 to 25 spots per quadrant
    ◦ Start at lower energy level and titrate up—more pigmented trabecular meshwork will require lower energy

- ° Avoid applying laser energy to the ciliary body band and Schwalbe's line
- ° For ALT
  - The laser applications should straddle the border of the pigmented and nonpigmented trabecular meshwork
  - Leave 1 to 2 spot diameters between adjacent laser applications
  - Titrate laser power until blanching of pigmented trabecular meshwork is seen without bubble formation
- ° For SLT
  - The laser applications should cover anterior scleral spur and pigmented and nonpigmented trabecular meshwork
  - Adjacent laser applications should be contiguous, but nonoverlapping
  - Titrate energy until fine "champagne bubbles" are seen over pigmented trabecular meshwork, then continue at level just below bubble-producing level
- ° For MLT/MDLT
  - Similar to SLT, but there is no visible tissue reaction

Postoperative Care and Follow-Up

- Recheck IOP 30 to 60 minutes after procedure
- No post-laser drops necessary (randomized controlled trial showed no difference in eyes that received post-SLT indomethacin 0.1% vs dexamethasone 0.1% vs no treatment)[33]
  - ° Some surgeons prefer a mild topical corticosteroid or nonsteroidal anti-inflammatory agent for 3 to 5 days
- Follow-up exam in 4 to 6 weeks to check IOP response

Complications

- IOP spike
- Transient anterior chamber inflammation
- Transient corneal endothelial changes (rare cases of permanent changes)[34]
- Formation of peripheral anterior synechiae (more so with continuous wave laser; eg, ALT)
- Insufficient reduction of IOP

Cyclophotocoagulation

Cyclophotocoagulation (CPC) involves the application of laser energy to the ciliary processes and ciliary body. The objective is to reduce aqueous humor production from the nonpigmented ciliary epithelium, thereby lowering the IOP. Early reports of transscleral CPC (TSCPC/TCP) described using a ruby laser (693 nm)[35] or Nd:YAG laser, but these have been superseded by the continuous wave, red diode laser (810 nm), which has greater absorption by uveal melanin compared to Nd:YAG and is more portable.[36] More recently, the use of pulsed laser has been described, which, like in pulsed-LTP, allows thermal relaxation and less adjacent tissue damage. Studies have demonstrated the efficacy of micropulse, transscleral, diode laser CPC (MP-TSCPC or MP-TCP) in lowering IOP in refractory glaucoma with an average of 40.1% to 59.9% reduction of IOP from baseline at 1 to 18 months postoperatively.[37-40] One study comparing continuous wave TSCPC to MP-TSCPC found similar efficacy between the 2 methods, but MP-TSCPC provided more consistent and predictable IOP-lowering effect and less ocular complications.[41]

In addition to the transscleral approach, CPC can be accomplished by applying laser directly to the ciliary body with the assistance of an endoscopic laser. Endoscopic cyclophotocoagulation (ECP) was first described by Uram in 1992 and involves directly applying laser to the ciliary body using an 18- to 20-gauge endoscope that also contains a light source and diode laser.[42] ECP can be performed via an anterior approach through a limbal incision or a posterior approach through the pars plana (ECP-plus) in combination with a pars plana vitrectomy.[43] In histopathological studies, ECP produced disruption of the ciliary body epithelium (the site of aqueous production and intended target for CPC), but less damage to other structures of the ciliary body when compared to eyes treated with TSCPC.[44] ECP has been shown to be effective in patients with refractory glaucoma with an average IOP reduction ranging from 34% to 66% at 12.9 to 24 months.[43,45,46] The safety and efficacy of ECP in combination with phacoemulsification has been reported in patients with nonrefractory glaucoma.[47-50] Phacoemulsification may also play a role in cases of plateau iris syndrome, especially in cases refractory to iridotomy and iridoplasty.[51,52] In this clinical setting, laser applications are used to produce contracture and posterior rotation of the ciliary processes.

Indications for TSCPC and MP-TSCPC

Due to risk of persistent inflammation, cystoid macular edema, hypotony, phthisis, and sympathetic ophthalmia, CPC has traditionally been reserved for refractory glaucoma with prior failed glaucoma procedures, eyes with minimal useful vision but elevated IOP, eyes with no visual potential but need pain relief, eyes with complicated glaucoma and conjunctival scarring, or situations that preclude incisional glaucoma surgery.[53] There is a lack of randomized controlled trials supporting its use as a primary procedure,[54] although its efficacy and relative safety as primary procedure has been described.[55,56]

Indications for Endoscopic Cyclophotocoagulation

Like MP-TSCPC and TSCPC, the indication for ECP has traditionally been the treatment of refractory glaucoma, but a number of studies support its use in nonrefractory glaucoma of varying severity and in eyes with good visual potential.[47-50] However, there is still a need for randomized controlled trials to assess the intermediate and long-term safety and efficacy of ECP for OAG and PAC.[57]

Laser Types

- TSCPC/TCP
  - Red diode, continuous wave (810 nm)
- MP-TSCPC/MP-TCP
  - Red diode, pulsed laser (810 nm)
- ECP
  - Red diode, continuous wave (810 nm)

Laser Settings

LASER	POWER/ENERGY	DURATION	SPOTS/DEGREES
TSCPC (diode, 810 nm)	400 to 1000 mW	0.1 sec	5 to 8 spots per quadrant (spaced about 1/2 width of G probe apart) for total of 15 to 40 applications over 180 to 360 degrees
MP-TSCPC (diode, 810 nm)	400 to 1000 mW	0.1 sec	Sweeping motions over 180 to 360 degrees
ECP (diode, 810 nm)	0.4 to 1.2 mJ	3 ns	Treatment through a corneal or pars plana incision Circumferential and anteroposterior extent of treatment dependent upon amount of effect desired

Procedure for TSCPC and MP-TSCPC

- Can be performed in office or operating room
- Confirm correct eye to be treated and that consent has been obtained

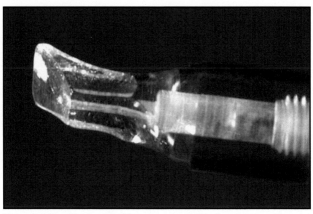

Figure 7-4. Tip of the G-probe. The narrower end of the footplate is positioned at the limbus during laser delivery.

- Anesthesia:
  - Operating room or office: retrobulbar/peribulbar block (50:50 mix of 0.75% bupivacaine and 2% lidocaine without epinephrine)
  - Operating room: general anesthesia is an option
- Instill 1 drop of proparacaine or tetracaine topical anesthetic
- May use an eyelid speculum
- Apply laser probe, to the sclera (make sure to orient proper edge of probe at the limbus)
  - Avoid 3:00 and 9:00 positions (long posterior ciliary arteries/nerves)
  - TSCPC
    - G probe (Iridex Corp): Titrate power in increments of 250 mW until popping sound is heard, then continue at setting just below this level
    - Apply 5 to 8 spots per quadrant (Figures 7-4 and 7-5)

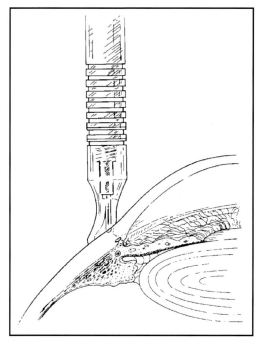

Figure 7-5. G-probe aligned at the limbus for laser delivery during diode laser cyclophotocoagulation. Note the orientation of the probe handle parallel with the visual axis. (Reproduced with permission from the American Academy of Ophthalmology.)

- ◦ MP-TSCPC
  - ▪ MicroPulse P3 probe (Iridex Corp): With a continuous sweeping motion, slide the probe over from 9:30 to 2:30, then 3:30 to 8:30 in a clockwise direction
- • Postprocedure (optional):
  - ◦ Posterior sub-Tenon's triamcinolone acetonide (40 mg in 1.0 mL)
  - ◦ Atropine 1% eye drop

Procedure for Endoscopic Cyclophotocoagulation

- Must be performed in the operating room
- Confirm correct eye to be treated and that consent has been obtained
- Dilate pupil preoperatively
- Anesthesia
  - Depending on the patient, retrobulbar, peribulbar, or topical
- Prepare the operative eye in sterile fashion and place eyelid speculum
- When combined with cataract surgery, perform cataract surgery first
- Inject viscoelastic to deepen the anterior chamber and expand the ciliary sulcus space
- Anterior approach (for phakic, pseudophakic, or aphakic eyes)
  - Utilize a 1.5 to 2.5 mm clear corneal incision to insert the ECP probe into the anterior chamber
- Posterior approach (for pseudophakic/aphakic eyes)
  - Perform a limited pars plana vitrectomy
  - Insert the ECP probe through a pars plana sclerotomy
- Apply laser to the ciliary processes (see previous Laser Settings section) by turning attention away from the microscope and to external monitor
  - Distance from the tip of the laser probe should be about 0.75 to 2.00 mm from ciliary process
  - Titrate power/duration until there is visible blanching/shrinkage of the ciliary process and lower the power/duration if there are visible bubbles or popping
- Remove viscoelastic from the anterior chamber (anterior approach)
- Ensure all wounds are watertight and close with suture if necessary
- May consider subconjunctival, posterior sub-Tenon's, or intracameral corticosteroid at the end of the procedure

Postoperative Care and Follow-Up

- Topical steroid (eg, prednisolone 1%) 4 to 6 times per day for 1 week, tapering over following 3 weeks
- Topical antibiotic 4 times a day for the first week
- Topical cycloplegia (eg, atropine 1%) 2 times a day for pain control

Complications

- TSCPC and MP-TSCPC:
  - Conjunctival burns
  - Pain
  - Hypotony
  - Inflammation
  - Hyphema
  - Corneal edema
  - Vision loss
  - Phthisis
  - Sympathetic ophthalmia (rare)
  - Need for retreatment
- ECP:
  - Same as TSCPC and MP-TSCPC, except for conjunctival burns
  - Zonular rupture
  - Endophthalmitis
  - Damage to the iris

Laser Suture Lysis

Laser suture lysis (LSL) is used to titrate filtration following trabeculectomy by selectively breaking the scleral flap sutures using laser energy through the intact conjunctiva. The sutures function to secure the flap and tamponade flow through the internal trabeculectomy ostium. In the immediate postoperative period, the tightness of the sutures determines the facility of aqueous outflow and the level of the IOP. Tight suturing of the scleral flap can help prevent postoperative hypotony but risks insufficient IOP lowering. As the eye heals, selective release of the flap sutures by breaking them with the laser reduces tension on the flap and results in enhancement of fluid flow and lowering of the IOP.[58,59] The timing of LSL and the number of sutures cut will depend on a variety of factors, including the use of antifibrotic agents, the size and configuration of the flap, the number of sutures placed at the time of surgery and their tightness, the desired target IOP, risk factors for complications related to hypotony, and the patient's postoperative course.

LSL can also be used to release the tube ligature of a nonvalved glaucoma drainage device, such as a Baerveldt implant (Johnson & Johnson Vision) or a Molteno implant (Nova Eye Medical). An absorbable (7-0 or 8-0 polyglactin) or nonabsorbable (7-0 or 8-0 polypropylene) suture can be used to constrict the tube to the point of complete luminal occlusion. The suture ligature is most often placed on the surface of the globe, beneath a corneal patch graft or posterior to a patch graft of any material. Laser energy can be used to relax or disrupt the suture, thereby releasing the tube constriction and initiating aqueous flow into the reservoir of the device.

Indications

- Trabeculectomy
  - ○ To enhance aqueous outflow and reduce the IOP by breaking 1 or more of the scleral flap anchoring sutures
- Glaucoma drainage device
  - ○ To release the occlusive ligature and initiate flow through the tube (Ritch suture lysis lens preferred, as the conical shape provides the best lid retraction for visualization of the posteriorly located suture)

Contraindications

- Shallow/flat anterior chamber
- Poor visualization of suture

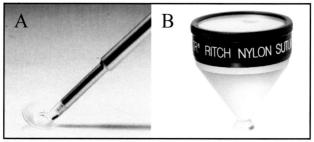

Figure 7-6. Hoskins (A) and Ritch (B) suture lysis lenses.

Laser Types

- Argon, continuous wave (488, 514, 532 nm)
- Green diode, continuous wave (532 nm)
- Krypton, continuous wave (647 nm; not absorbed by blood)

Laser Settings

LASER	POWER	DURATION	SPOT SIZE
Argon or diode	200 to 1000 mW	0.05 sec	50 to 75 μm
Krypton	150 to 500 mW	0.05 sec	50 to 75 μm

Lenses

- Hoskins suture lysis (Figure 7-6A)
- Ritch suture lysis (Figure 7-6B)
- Mandelkorn suture lysis

Procedure

- Confirm correct eye to be treated and that consent has been obtained
- Instill 1 drop of proparacaine or tetracaine topical anesthetic and 1 drop of 2.5% phenylephrine to constrict conjunctival vessels
- Place LSL lens over the suture, compressing the conjunctiva against the sclera to blanch blood vessels and obtain better visualization
- Apply laser until suture is lysed (see previous Laser Settings section)
  - Trabeculectomy
    - Start with low power (200 to 300 mW) and increase as needed to achieve visible disruption of the suture
    - In general, higher power will be required for more poorly visualized sutures
  - Glaucoma drainage device
    - Multiple laser applications are often required to loosen/break the ligature
    - Higher laser power (600 to 800 mW) is generally needed to release a ligature that is beneath a corneal patch graft
    - Visible breakage of a polyglactin ligature is often difficult to visualize, so it is important to check intermittently for softening of the globe

Postoperative Care and Follow-Up

- Recheck IOP following procedure
- Continue any postoperative drops as appropriate
- Follow-up in 1 week to recheck IOP

Complications

- Conjunctival burn
- Shallow/flat anterior chamber
- Conjunctival perforation/leak
- Hypotony
- Malignant glaucoma

Lens Choices

- ocularinc.com
- accutome.com

LENS	INDICATIONS	CONTACT DIAMETER	IMAGE MAGNIFICATION	LASER SPOT MAGNIFICATION
Abraham iridectomy	LPI, PICP	15.5 mm	1.6x	0.63x
Wise iridotomy	LPI, PICP	15.5 mm	2.6x	0.38x
Pollack iridotomy/gonio	LPI	15 mm	1.5x	0.65x
Ritch trabeculoplasty	LTP, SLT	18 mm	1.4x	0.71x
Goldmann 3-mirror lens	LTP, SLT	15 to 20 mm	0.93x	1.08x
Latina	SLT	14.5 to 18.0 mm	1.0x	1.0x
Hoskins suture lysis	LSL	3.0 mm	1.2x	0.83x
Ritch suture lysis	LSL	5.7 mm	1.0x	1.0x
Mandelkorn suture lysis	LSL	5.6 mm	1.32x	0.76x

LPI = laser peripheral iridotomy; LSL = laser suture lysis; LTP = laser trabeculoplasty; PICP = peripheral iris contraction procedure; SLT = selective laser trabeculoplasty.

REFERENCES

1. How AC, Baskaran M, Kumar RS, et al. Changes in anterior segment morphology after laser peripheral iridotomy: an anterior segment optical coherence tomography study. *Ophthalmology*. 2012;119(7):1383-1387.

2. Lee KS, Sung KR, Shon K, Sun JH, Lee JR. Longitudinal changes in anterior segment parameters after laser peripheral iridotomy assessed by anterior segment optical coherence tomography. *Invest Ophthalmol Vis Sci*. 2013;54(5):3166-3170.

3. Jiang Y, Chang DS, Zhu H, et al. Longitudinal changes of angle configuration in primary angle-closure suspects: the zhongshan angle-closure prevention trial. *Ophthalmology*. 2014;121(9):1699-1705.

4. He M, Friedman DS, Ge J, et al. Laser peripheral iridotomy in primary angle-closure suspects: biometric and gonioscopic outcomes: the Liwan Eye Study. *Ophthalmology*. 2007;114(3):494-500.

5. Lee KS, Sung KR, Kang SY, et al. Residual anterior chamber angle closure in narrow-angle eyes following laser peripheral iridotomy: anterior segment optical coherence tomography quantitative study. *Jpn J Ophthalmol*. 2011;55(3):213-219.

6. Baskaran M, Yang E, Trikha S, et al. Residual angle closure one year after laser peripheral iridotomy in primary angle closure suspects. *Am J Ophthalmol*. 2017;183:111-117.

7. Michelessi M, Lindsley K. Peripheral iridotomy for pigmentary glaucoma. *Cochrane Database Syst Rev*. 2016;2:Cd005655.

8. Vera V, Nagi A, Belovay GW, Varma DK, Ahmed II. Dysphotopsia after temporal versus superior laser peripheral iridaotomy: a prospective randomized paired eye trial. *Am J Ophthalmol*. 2014;157(5):929-935.

9. Srinivasan K, Zebardast N, Krishnamurthy P, et al. Comparison of new visual disturbances after superior versus nasal/temporal laser peripheral iridotomy: a prospective randomized trial. *Ophthalmology*. 2018;125(3):345-351.

10. Lai JSM, Tham CCY, Chua JKH, Lam DSC. Immediate diode laser peripheral iridoplasty as treatment of acute attack of primary angle closure glaucoma: a preliminary study. *J Glaucoma*. 2001;10(2):89-94.

11. Ritch R, Tham CC, Lam DS. Argon laser peripheral iridoplasty (ALPI): an update. *Surv Ophthalmol*. 2007;52(3):279-288.

12. Ritch R, Tham CC, Lam DS. Long-term success of argon laser peripheral iridoplasty in the management of plateau iris syndrome. *Ophthalmology*. 2004;111(1):104-108.

13. Peterson JR, Anderson JW, Blieden LS, et al. Long-term outcome of argon laser peripheral iridoplasty in the management of plateau iris syndrome eyes. *J Glaucoma*. 2017;26(9):780-786.

14. Narayanaswamy A, Baskaran M, Perera SA, et al. Argon laser peripheral iridoplasty for primary angle-closure glaucoma: a randomized controlled trial. *Ophthalmology*. 2016;123(3):514-521.

15. Wise JB, Witter SL. Argon laser therapy for open-angle glaucoma. A pilot study. *Arch Ophthalmol.* 1979;97(2):319-322.

16. Glaucoma Laser Trial Research Group. The Glaucoma Laser Trial (GLT) and glaucoma laser trial follow-up study: 7. Results. *Am J Ophthalmol.* 1995;120(6):718-731.

17. Latina MA, Sibayan SA, Shin DH, Noecker RJ, Marcellino G. Q-switched 532-nm Nd:YAG laser trabeculoplasty (selective laser trabeculoplasty): a multicenter, pilot, clinical study. *Ophthalmology.* 1998;105(11):2082-2088; discussion 2089-2090.

18. McAlinden C. Selective laser trabeculoplasty (SLT) vs other treatment modalities for glaucoma: systematic review. *Eye (Lond).* 2014;28(3):249-258.

19. Juzych MS, Chopra V, Banitt MR, et al. Comparison of long-term outcomes of selective laser trabeculoplasty versus argon laser trabeculoplasty in open-angle glaucoma. *Ophthalmology.* 2004;111(10):1853-1859.

20. Nagar M, Ogunyomade A, O'Brart DP, Howes F, Marshall J. A randomised, prospective study comparing selective laser trabeculoplasty with latanoprost for the control of intraocular pressure in ocular hypertension and open angle glaucoma. *Br J Ophthalmol.* 2005;89(11):1413-1417.

21. Gracner T, Falez M, Gracner B, Pahor D. [Long-term follow-up of selective laser trabeculoplasty in primary open-angle glaucoma]. *Klin Monbl Augenheilkd.* 2006;223(9):743-747.

22. Weinand FS, Althen F. Long-term clinical results of selective laser trabeculoplasty in the treatment of primary open angle glaucoma. *Eur J Ophthalmol.* 2006;16(1):100-104.

23. Bovell AM, Damji KF, Hodge WG, et al. Long term effects on the lowering of intraocular pressure: selective laser or argon laser trabeculoplasty? *Can J Ophthalmol.* 2011;46(5):408-413.

24. Hodge WG, Damji KF, Rock W, et al. Baseline IOP predicts selective laser trabeculoplasty success at 1 year post-treatment: results from a randomised clinical trial. *Br J Ophthalmol.* 2005;89(9):1157-1160.

25. Chun M, Gracitelli CP, Lopes FS, et al. Selective laser trabeculoplasty for early glaucoma: analysis of success predictors and adjusted laser outcomes based on the untreated fellow eye. *BMC Ophthalmol.* 2016;16(1):206.

26. Pillunat KR, Spoerl E, Elfes G, Pillunat LE. Preoperative intraocular pressure as a predictor of selective laser trabeculoplasty efficacy. *Acta Ophthalmol.* 2016;94(7):692-696.

27. Birt CM. Selective laser trabeculoplasty retreatment after prior argon laser trabeculoplasty: 1-year results. *Can J Ophthalmol.* 2007;42(5):715-719.

28. Hong BK, Winer JC, Martone JF, et al. Repeat selective laser trabeculoplasty. *J Glaucoma.* 2009;18(3):180-183.

29. Ayala M. Intraocular pressure reduction after initial failure of selective laser trabeculoplasty (SLT). *Graefes Arch Clin Exp Ophthalmol.* 2014;252(2):315-320.

30. Polat J, Grantham L, Mitchell K, Realini T. Repeatability of selective laser trabeculoplasty. *Br J Ophthalmol.* 2016;100(10):1437-1441.

31. Francis BA, Loewen N, Hong B, et al. Repeatability of selective laser trabeculoplasty for open-angle glaucoma. *BMC Ophthalmol.* 2016;16:128.

32. Ingvoldstad D, Krishna R, Willoughby L. Micropulse diode laser trabeculoplasty versus argon laser trabeculoplasty in the treatment of open angle glaucoma. *Invest Ophthalmol Vis Sci.* 2005;46(123).

33. De Keyser M, De Belder M, De Groot V. Randomized prospective study of the use of anti-inflammatory drops after selective laser trabeculoplasty. *J Glaucoma.* 2017;26(2):e22-e29.

34. Liu ET, Seery LS, Arosemena A, Lamba T, Chaya CJ. Corneal edema and keratitis following selective laser trabeculoplasty. *Am J Ophthalmol Case Rep.* 2017;6:48-51.

35. Beckman H, Kinoshita A, Rota AN, Sugar HS. Transscleral ruby laser irradiation of the ciliary body in the treatment of intractable glaucoma. *Trans Am Acad Ophthalmol Otolaryngol.* 1972;76(2):423-436.

36. Gaasterland DE, Pollack IP. Initial experience with a new method of laser transscleral cyclophotocoagulation for ciliary ablation in severe glaucoma. *Trans Am Ophthalmol Soc.* 1992;90:225-246.

37. Tan AM, Chockalingam M, Aquino MC, et al. Micropulse transscleral diode laser cyclophotocoagulation in the treatment of refractory glaucoma. *Clin Exp Ophthalmol.* 2010;38(3):266-272.

38. Kuchar S, Moster MR, Reamer CB, Waisbourd M. Treatment outcomes of micropulse transscleral cyclophotocoagulation in advanced glaucoma. *Lasers Med Sci.* 2016;31(2):393-396.

39. Emanuel ME, Grover DS, Fellman RL, et al. Micropulse cyclophotocoagulation: initial results in refractory glaucoma. *J Glaucoma.* 2017;26(8):726-729.

40. Williams AL, Moster MR, Rahmatnejad K, et al. Clinical efficacy and safety profile of micropulse transscleral cyclophotocoagulation in refractory glaucoma. *J Glaucoma.* 2018;27(5):445-449.

41. Aquino MC, Barton K, Tan AM, et al. Micropulse versus continuous wave transscleral diode cyclophotocoagulation in refractory glaucoma: a randomized exploratory study. *Clin Exp Ophthalmol.* 2015;43(1):40-46.

42. Uram M. Ophthalmic laser microendoscope endophotocoagulation. *Ophthalmology.* 1992;99(12):1829-1832.

43. Tan JC, Francis BA, Noecker R, et al. Endoscopic cyclophotocoagulation and pars plana ablation (ecp-plus) to treat refractory glaucoma. *J Glaucoma.* 2016;25(3):e117-e122.

44. Pantcheva MB, Kahook MY, Schuman JS, Noecker RJ. Comparison of acute structural and histopathological changes in human autopsy eyes after endoscopic cyclophotocoagulation and trans-scleral cyclophotocoagulation. *Br J Ophthalmol.* 2007;91(2):248-252.

45. Chen J, Cohn RA, Lin SC, Cortes AE, Alvarado JA. Endoscopic photocoagulation of the ciliary body for treatment of refractory glaucomas. *Am J Ophthalmol.* 1997;124(6):787-796.

46. Murthy GJ, Murthy PR, Murthy KR, Kulkarni VV, Murthy KR. A study of the efficacy of endoscopic cyclophotocoagulation for the treatment of refractory glaucomas. *Indian J Ophthalmol.* 2009;57(2):127-132.

47. Lima FE, Carvalho DM, Avila MP. [Phacoemulsification and endoscopic cyclophotocoagulation as primary surgical procedure in coexisting cataract and glaucoma]. *Arq Bras Oftalmol.* 2010;73(5):419-422.

48. Lindfield D, Ritchie RW, Griffiths MF. "Phaco-ECP": combined endoscopic cyclophotocoagulation and cataract surgery to augment medical control of glaucoma. *BMJ Open.* 2012;2(3):e000578.

49. Francis BA, Berke SJ, Dustin L, Noecker R. Endoscopic cyclophotocoagulation combined with phacoemulsification versus phacoemulsification alone in medically controlled glaucoma. *J Cataract Refract Surg.* 2014;40(8):1313-1321.

50. Siegel MJ, Boling WS, Faridi OS, et al. Combined endoscopic cyclophotocoagulation and phacoemulsification versus phacoemulsification alone in the treatment of mild to moderate glaucoma. *Clin Exp Ophthalmol.* 2015;43(6):531-539.

51. Francis BA, Pouw A, Jenkins D, et al. Endoscopic cycloplasty (ECPL) and lens extraction in the treatment of severe plateau iris syndrome. *J Glaucoma.* 2016;25(3):e128-e133.

52. Hollander DA, Pennesi ME, Alvarado JA. Management of plateau iris syndrome with cataract extraction and endoscopic cyclophotocoagulation. *Exp Eye Res.* 2017;158:190-194.

53. Pastor SA, Singh K, Lee DA, et al. Cyclophotocoagulation: a report by the American Academy of Ophthalmology. *Ophthalmology.* 2001;108(11):2130-2138.

54. Michelessi M, Bicket AK, Lindsley K. Cyclodestructive procedures for non-refractory glaucoma. *Cochrane Database Syst Rev.* 2018;4:Cd009313.

55. Grueb M, Rohrbach JM, Bartz-Schmidt KU, Schlote T. Transscleral diode laser cyclophotocoagulation as primary and secondary surgical treatment in primary open-angle and pseudoexfoliatve glaucoma. Long-term clinical outcomes. *Graefes Arch Clin Exp Ophthalmol.* 2006;244(10):1293-1299.

56. Gorsler I, Thieme H, Meltendorf C. Cyclophotocoagulation and cyclocryocoagulation as primary surgical procedures for open-angle glaucoma. *Graefes Arch Clin Exp Ophthalmol.* 2015;253(12):2273-2277.

57. Toth M, Shah A, Hu K, Bunce C, Gazzard G. Endoscopic cyclophotocoagulation (ECP) for open angle glaucoma and primary angle closure. *Cochrane Database Syst Rev.* 2019;2:Cd012741.

58. Savage JA, Condon GP, Lytle RA, Simmons RJ. Laser suture lysis after trabeculectomy. *Ophthalmology.* 1988;95(12):1631-1638.

59. Morinelli EN, Sidoti PA, Heuer DK, et al. Laser suture lysis after mitomycin C trabeculectomy. *Ophthalmology.* 1996;103(2):306-314.

8

Medical Management of Glaucoma

Sara J. Coulon, MD
and Murray Fingeret, OD

INTRODUCTION

The goal of currently available glaucoma therapy is to lower the intraocular pressure (IOP) to a target range thought to likely prevent further optic nerve damage. This target is individualized, adjustable throughout the course of treatment, and is usually based on the following: maximum IOP, stage of disease, observed rate of progression, life expectancy of the patient, and other known risks (ie, history of disc hemorrhage, thin pachymetry, family history of glaucoma). The clinician must decide how to achieve this goal—medically, with laser, or surgically—considering the impact of treatment vs disease progression on the quality of life of the patient.

Initial treatment of most forms of glaucoma includes the use of topical medications. Other options include selective laser trabeculoplasty, cataract surgery performed with or without a microinvasive glaucoma surgery and, in advanced cases, traditional glaucoma surgery. Approximately 50% of individuals will

Panarelli JF, ed.
The Pocket Guide to Glaucoma (pp 119-140).
© 2022 Taylor & Francis Group.

require more than 1 agent or modality during their lifetime of care. This chapter will concentrate on the role of medical therapy to reduce IOP with the goal of preventing visual decline.

MEDICATION CLASSES

Ocular hypotensive agents are divided into classes based on their mechanisms of action: prostaglandin analogues (PGAs), adrenergic agents (beta-adrenergic antagonists, adrenergic agonists), carbonic anhydrase inhibitors (CAIs), parasympathomimetic agents (direct-acting and indirect-acting), rho-kinase agents, and combination agents. Table 8-1 provides a timetable of discovery for each class. Table 8-2 lists each class with its recommended dosing, mechanism of action, and side effects. Brand names and available concentrations of medicines are listed in Table 8-3.

Prostaglandin Analogues

PGAs are commonly used as first-line agents. These drugs lower IOP by increasing outflow via the uveoscleral pathway. There are 4 analogues in clinical use: latanoprost (first PGA introduced in 1996), bimatoprost, travoprost, and tafluprost (preservative-free). All are dosed once nightly and are less efficacious when used twice daily. They reduce IOP by 30% to 35% with few systemic or ocular side effects.[1,2] Adverse effects include iris darkening (irreversible); conjunctival hyperemia, hypertrichosis, trichiasis, distichiasis, periocular skin irritation (reversible); periorbital fat atrophy, development of enophthalmos[3] (unclear if reversible); cystoid macula edema, reactivation of herpetic keratitis, and development of nongranulamatous anterior uveitis.[2] Of note, some patients may respond better to 1 agent in this class than to another, but clinicians should trial each agent for 4 to 6 weeks before switching.

Table 8-1. Year of Discovery

CLASS	APPROVED	EXAMPLE	DOSAGE	NOTES
Miotics	1875	Pilocarpine	QID	Rarely used
Beta-blockers	1978	Timolol	BID	Often only used in the morning
Topical carbonic anhydrase inhibitors	1994	Dorzolamide	TID	Commonly used BID in combination with other medications
Prostaglandins	1996	Latanoprost	QHS	
Alpha-2-agonists	1996	Brimonidine	TID	Commonly used BID in combination with other medications
Fixed combination	1998	Cosopt	BID	
Rho-kinase inhibitors	2017	Netarsudil	QD	

BID = 2 times a day; QD = 1 time a day; QHS = every day at bedtime; QID = 4 times a day; TID = 3 times a day.

Table 8-2. Topical Glaucoma Drops, Mechanisms of Action, and Side Effects

NAME	DOSING	MECHANISM OF ACTION	OCULAR SIDE EFFECTS	SYSTEMIC SIDE EFFECTS
PROSTAGLANDIN ANALOGUES				
Latanoprost Travoprost Bimatoprost Tafluprost (PF)	Once daily	Increases uveoscleral outflow	Increased iris pigmentation Hypertrichosis Keratitis Anterior uveitis Conjunctival hyperemia CME	Flu-like symptoms Headache Joint/muscle pain
BETA-ADRENERGIC ANTAGONISTS				
Timolol maleate Timolol hemihydrate Levobunolol Metipranolol Carteolol	Solutions: 1 to 2 times daily Gels: once daily	Decreases aqueous production	Blurring Irritation Corneal anesthesia Punctate keratitis Exacerbation of mysasthenia gravis	Bradycardia Bronchospasm Lowered blood pressure CNS depression Masked symptoms of hypoglycemia

(continued)

NAME	DOSING	MECHANISM OF ACTION	OCULAR SIDE EFFECTS	SYSTEMIC SIDE EFFECTS
Betaxolol (selective B1)	2 times daily	Decreases aqueous production	Same as previous	Lower risk of pulmonary complications
ALPHA-2-ADRENERGIC AGONISTS				
Apraclonidine	2 to 3 times daily	Decreases aqueous production	Irritation Ocular allergy Conjunctival blanching Follicular conjunctivitis Ocular ache Miosis	Hypotension Fatigue Vasovagal attack
Brimonidine tartrate 0.2%	2 to 3 times daily	Decreases aqueous production	Blurring Foreign body sensation Dryness Ocular allergy	Headache Fatigue Depression Syncope Anxiety

Table 8-2. Topical Glaucoma Drops, Mechanisms of Action, and Side Effects (continued)

(continued)

Table 8-2. Topical Glaucoma Drops, Mechanisms of Action, and Side Effects (continued)

NAME	DOSING	MECHANISM OF ACTION	OCULAR SIDE EFFECTS	SYSTEMIC SIDE EFFECTS
Brimonidine tartrate 0.1% in Purite	2 to 3 times daily	Decreases aqueous production	Less allergy than previous	Less fatigue and depression than previous
Carbonic Anhydrase Inhibitors				
Oral acetazolamide	250 mg 2 to 4 times daily 500 mg 2 times daily	Decreases aqueous production	None	Acidosis Depression Malaise Paresthesias Lethargy Diarrhea Renal stones Loss of libido Altered taste Hypokalemia

(continued)

Table 8-2. Topical Glaucoma Drops, Mechanisms of Action, and Side Effects (continued)

NAME	DOSING	MECHANISM OF ACTION	OCULAR SIDE EFFECTS	SYSTEMIC SIDE EFFECTS
Oral methazolamide	25 mg 2 to 3 times daily 50 mg 2 to 3 times daily	Decreases aqueous production	None	Less renal complications than previous
Topical dorzolamide	2 to 3 times daily	Decreases aqueous production	Stinging Blurred vision Keratitis Conjunctivitis	Bitter taste Less likely to cause systemic complications
Topical brinzolamide	2 to 3 times daily	Decreases aqueous production	Same as previous with less stinging	Same as previous
PARASYMPATHOMIMETICS				
Pilocarpine (direct-acting)	2 to 4 times daily	Increases trabecular outflow	Keratitis Miosis Brow ache	Increased salivation Abdominal cramps

(continued)

Table 8-2. Topical Glaucoma Drops, Mechanisms of Action, and Side Effects (continued)

NAME	DOSING	MECHANISM OF ACTION	OCULAR SIDE EFFECTS	SYSTEMIC SIDE EFFECTS
			Angle-closure potential	
			Myopia	
			Retinal detachment	
Echothiophate (indirect-acting)	1 to 2 times daily	Increases trabecular outflow	Intense miosis	Same as previous
			Iris pigment cyst	Anesthesia risk of prolonged recovery
			Myopia	
			Retinal detachment	
			Pseudopemphigoid	

Adapted from Girkin GA, Bhorade AM, Crowston JG, et al. Medical management of glaucoma. In: Girkin GA, Bhorade AM, Crowston JG, et al. *2019-2020 BCSC (Basic and Clinical Science Course), Section 10: Glaucoma.* American Academy of Ophthalmology; 2019:169-186.

Color coded by typical commercial top color.

CME = cystoid macular edema; CNS = central nervous system; PF = preservative free.

Table 8-3. Brand Names and Concentrations

BRAND NAME/MANUFACTURER	GENERIC NAME	CONCENTRATION/BOTTLE SIZE
BETA-BLOCKERS GENERIC (MULTIPLE MANUFACTURERS)		
Betimol/Vistakon	Timolol hemihydrate	0.25% / 5 mL
		0.5% / 5 mL, 10 mL, 15 mL
Betopic-S/Alcon	Betaxolol HCL	0.25% / 2.5 mL, 5 mL, 10 mL, 15 mL
Istalol/Ista	Timolol maleate	0.5% / 5 mL
Betagan/Allergan	Levobunolol	0.25% / 5 mL, 10 mL, 15 mL
		0.5% / 5 mL, 10 mL, 15 mL
Timoptic (PF)/Aton Pharma	Timolol maleate	0.25% / unit dose
		0.5% / unit dose
Timoptic-XE/Aton Pharma	Timolol maleate	0.25% / 2.5 mL, 5 mL
		0.5% / 2.5 mL, 5 mL
PROSTAGLANDIN ANALOGUES		
Lumigan/Allergan	Bimatoprost	0.01% / 2.5 mL, 5 mL, 7.5 mL
Rescula	Unoprostone	0.15% / 2.5 mL, 5 mL

(continued)

Table 8-3. Brand Names and Concentrations (continued)

BRAND NAME/MANUFACTURER	GENERIC NAME	CONCENTRATION/BOTTLE SIZE
Travatan Z/Alcon	Travoprost	0.004% / 2.5 mL, 5 mL
Generic	Latanoprost	0.005% / 2.5 mL
Zioptan/Merck	Tafluprost	2.5 mL
PROSTAGLANDIN + NITRIC OXIDE		
Vyzulta/Bausch + Lomb	Latanoprostene bunod	0.024% / 5 mL
ALPHA AGONISTS		
Generic	Brimonidine	0.1%, 0.15% / 5 mL, 10 mL, 15 mL
Alphagan P/Allergan	Brimonidine	0.1%, 0.15% / 5 mL, 10 mL, 15 mL
Iopidine/Alcon	Apraclonidine	0.5% / 5 mL, 10 mL
		1% / unit dose
CARBONIC ANHYDRASE INHIBITORS		
Azopt/Alcon	Brinzolamide	1% / 5 mL, 10 mL, 15 mL
Generic; multiple manufacturers	Dorzolamide	2% / 5 mL, 10 mL

(continued)

Table 8-3. Brand Names and Concentrations (continued)		
BRAND NAME/MANUFACTURER	GENERIC NAME	CONCENTRATION/BOTTLE SIZE
RHO-KINASE INHIBITORS		
Rhopressa/Aerie	Netarusdil	0.02% / 2.5 mL
COMBINATION GLAUCOMA MEDICATIONS		
Combigan/Allergan	Brimonidine/timolol	0.2%, 0.5% / 5 mL, 10 mL
Simbrinza/Alcon	Brinzolamide/brimonidine	1%, 0.2% / 8 mL
Cosopt PF/Merck Generic	Dorzolamide/timolol	2%, 0.5% / 5 mL, 10 mL
Timolol-dorzolamide	Dorzolamide/timolol	2%, 0.5% / 5 mL, 10 mL
Generic; multiple manufacturers		

PF = preservative-free.

Latanoprostene bunod is a newer PGA that was approved in November 2017, and it has a dual mechanism of action. The molecule is metabolized to latanoprost acid and utanediol mononitrate (a nitric-oxide donating moiety), which work to improve aqueous outflow via the uveoslceral pathway and trabecular meshwork (TM), respectively. It is used once per day and has a side effect profile similar to latanoprost. It has shown approximately 1.23 mm Hg greater IOP lowering as compared to latanoprost.[4-6]

Adrenergic Agents

Beta-Adrenergic Antagonists

Topical beta-blockers have a long history of use, going back to their introduction in 1976.[7] These drugs lower IOP by reducing aqueous humor secretion by inhibiting cyclic adenosine monophosphate production in the ciliary epithelium. There are currently 6 agents in clinical use: betaxolol (cardioselective; targets beta-1 receptors), carteolol, levobunolol, metipranolol, timolol maleate, and timolol hemihydrate (nonselective; targets beta-1 and beta-2 receptors). They reduce IOP by 20% to 30%.[7] Dosage is approved as twice per day, but beta-blockers have been shown to have less effect on aqueous secretion during nocturnal hours due to already reduced production during sleep[8]; for this reason, many clinicians prescribe the agent once a day in the morning. Betaxolol, the only cardioselective agent named above, is considered less effective in lowering IOP than the other nonselective agents but may play a role in patients with lung disease.

Systemic adverse effects from beta-blockers include bronchospasm, bradycardia, lethargy, depression, masking of hypoglyemic symptoms, reduced libido, and alteration of serum lipids; ocular side effects include corneal anesthesia and punctate keratitis. These drugs are typically not used in patients with asthma, chronic obstructive pulmonary disease, or cardiac disease. Also, interestingly, tachyphylaxis and/or short-term escape is sometimes seen with topical beta-blocker use, whereby the efficacy of the medication is reduced over time.[9]

Alpha-2-Adrenergic Agonists

Alpha-2 selective agonists lower IOP by reducing aqueous humor production via activation of the alpha-2-adrenoceptor coupled to an inhibitory G-protein. There are 2 agents available. Brimonidine tartrate is the most commonly used, whereas apraclonidine hydrochloride is rarely used long-term due to the high risk of tachyphylaxis and blepharoconjunctivitis. Alpha agonists reduce IOP by approximately 20% and are additive to other agents.[10] Similar to beta-blockers, they do not reduce IOP during the nocturnal hours.[11] Systemic side effects include dry mouth and lethargy. Of note, these agents should not be used in infants and young children because of the risk of central nervous system depression.[10] Ocular side effects include follicular conjunctivitis, contact blepharodermatitis, conjunctival vasoconstriction, and rarely, granulomatous anterior uveitis.

Though not typically used for long-term glaucoma therapy, apraclonidine is frequently used before laser iridotomy, laser trabeculoplasty, and Nd:YAG laser capsulotomy to abate acute IOP spikes after these procedures.

Carbonic Anhydrase Inhibitors

CAIs lower IOP by decreasing aqueous humor production via inhibition of ciliary epithelial carbonic anhydrase. Initially, only systemic CAIs (acetazolamide, methazolamide) were available; they provide excellent IOP reduction but have several potential side effects, including metabolic acidosis, hypokalemia, metallic taste, loss of energy, anorexia, weight loss, development of kidney stones, paresthesias, aplastic anemia, and risk of sickle cell crisis.[12] Methazolamide is considered safer for patients with renal insufficiency, as it is metabolized by the liver. Topical carbonic anhydrase agents were introduced in 1994, with the rationale of obtaining IOP-lowering effects without the systemic problems associated with this class.[13] There are currently 2 topical CAIs in clinical use: dorzolamide and brinzolamide. Topical CAIs reduce IOP by approximately 18% to 20%[13] with common side effects including bitter taste, transient blurred vision, and burning with instillation due to the low pH.[14] There is a small risk of corneal decompensation with use of topical CAIs in eyes with compromised corneal endothelial cell function. Topical CAIs show similar efficacy whether used alone or as an addition to other agents.[14,15] Topical CAI dosage is 3 times daily when used alone but often dosed 2 times daily when combined with other agents.

Parasympathomimetic Agents

Cholinergic agents have been used to reduce IOP for more than 100 years. This class is divided into direct-acting cholinergic agents and indirect-acting cholinesterase inhibitors: pilocarpine and echothiophate iodide, respectively. Both agents reduce IOP by causing contraction of the longitudinal ciliary muscle fibers that insert onto the scleral spur and TM, causing increased outflow facility. Pilocarpine is available in concentrations from 1% to 8%, with 1%, 2%, and 4% being the most often used concentrations.[16] Pilocarpine reduces IOP by 15% to 25%, and dosing ranges from 2 to 4 times daily. Echothiophate iodide is very rarely used; it can cause decreased metabolism of succinylcholine, a muscle relaxant used in general anesthesia, resulting in prolonged respiratory paralysis. Miotics have significant ocular side effects, such as blurred vision, brow ache, headache, induced myopia, and dim vision, that make these medicines intolerable for many patients. There have also been reports of reactivation of uveitis or development of retinal detachments with the use of miotics.[17] Pilocarpine is safer than echothiophate systemically; thus, while rarely used, currently accepted indications for use include in plateau iris syndrome patients or to blunt IOP spikes from strenuous physical activity in pigmentary glaucoma patients.

Rho-Kinase Agents

Rho-kinase inhibitors (netarsudil) are a newer class of medication, first introduced in 2017. They reduce IOP by targeting the TM to reduce its stiffness.[18] The medication targets the TM at the cellular level, inhibiting the creation of stress fibers to enhance

TM outflow.[18] The medication reduces IOP approximately 20% to 22% and is dosed once per day. Side effects include hyperemia, development of small hemorrhages at the limbal border, and corneal verticilatta.[19] Its efficacy is greater when the IOP is in the mid-20s and lower, which is unusual, as most agents show greater efficacy with higher IOP.[20] It appears to be safe systemically, and work is ongoing to understand its additivity to other agents.

Combination Agents

Fixed-combination agents are invaluable in the medical management of glaucoma, as they can improve patient adherence and reduce cost. Currently available combination agents include timolol-dorzolamide, timolol-brimonidine, brimondine-brinzolamide (dosed twice daily); and netarsudil-latanoprost (dosed once daily). These agents have a side effect profile and efficacy that matches the individual agents found in the combination. Some clinicians now use fixed-combination agents as their second-line agent, after the use of PGAs.

Newer Drug Delivery Systems

Adherence to multiple topical medications is understandably difficult. There is ongoing research regarding new drug delivery systems, such as drug depot subconjunctival inserts, intravitreal inserts, punctal plugs, and contact lenses, that could provide more convenient medical options for glaucoma treatment.

BEGINNING TREATMENT

All the medications previously listed are reasonable choices for first-line therapy. PGAs are typically used as primary therapy due to excellent ability to lower IOP, favorable safety profile, once-daily dosing regimen, and affordability. However, there are times where other medications may be more suitable, and this is based on individual patient needs.

Depending upon the class of medication, anywhere from 10% to 20% of individuals will be nonresponders (< 15% IOP reduction).[21] In this case, the clinician must consider changing and/or adding classes of medications, as well as laser and/or incisional surgery. Before this is done, however, it is important to ask patients about how often they use their drops, problems with eye drop instillation, side effects, and trouble with cost to better elucidate true treatment failure from poor adherence.

THE MONOCULAR TRIAL: WHERE HAS IT GONE?

The monocular trial is of historic interest since, until recently, it was often used when therapy was initiated. With the monocular trial, topical therapy was started in 1 eye, using the nontreated eye as a control. The medication was used for a few weeks and IOP was evaluated in both eyes, examining the reduction as well as side effects. A substantial decrease in the treated eye would indicate therapeutic success, with the medication then used in both eyes. There have been reports in the literature demonstrating that the monocular trial is not a useful tool in predicting if a medication will be effective because the 2 eyes do not work in sync (1 eye may rise or fall differently from the other) and the therapeutic response in 1 eye does not predict the response in the other.[22-27]

Many clinicians now recommend checking at least 1 untreated IOP pressure readings before therapy is initiated (preferably at different times of the day) and then starting the medication in both eyes. If a therapeutic response is not seen, it is recommended to recheck the IOP again a few weeks later before moving on to a different medication.

FOLLOW-UP VISITS

The goal of therapy is to reduce the IOP to a range that will prevent further structural and/or functional deterioration. The target IOP is a range of pressures based upon the person's history, extent of damage (optic nerve/retinal nerve fiber layer [RNFL] and visual field status) and level of the IOP (Figure 8-1). Other factors include the person's age as well as ocular and family history. The greater the amount of damage and higher the IOP, the lower the IOP should be to stabilize the condition. It is easier to obtain significant IOP reduction when the IOP starts high. IOP in the teens often allows only 2 to 4 mm Hg of reduction. The way to know if the person is controlled (and at the target IOP) is by evaluating for change in structural and functional tests over time (Figure 8-2). The caveat is that it takes approximately 5 tests (optical coherence tomography [OCT], visual fields) before the statistical software provided with most devices is robust enough to ascertain if stability is present.

The analysis and role of OCT and visual fields will be discussed in greater detail in later chapters, but 1 important question to consider is when to perform these tests. Traditionally, diagnostic testing was done on a yearly basis, meaning it could take several years before progression was recognized. Work by Chauhan et al and Crabb et al showed that front-loading tests is useful to detect change and thus allow earlier intervention.[28,29] Approximately 10% of newly diagnosed individuals will show rapid progression that will only be discovered by increasing the number of tests performed after the diagnosis is made.[21] The authors recommend testing with OCT and visual fields at the time of diagnosis and at 6, 12, 18, and 24 months, which is similar to recommendations by the European Glaucoma Society (which recommends 3 tests done for the first 2 years after diagnosis).[30] By 2 years, the 5 tests performed provide an idea of stability. If there is concern for progression, adjustment to target IOP and

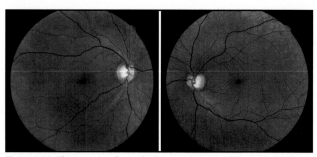

Figure 8-1A. This is a case of a newly diagnosed 70-year-old individual with primary open-angle glaucoma; damage is worse in the left eye. An inferior wedge RNFL defect is seen in the right eye with an average RNFL of 70 μm in a large optic disc (2.78 mm²).

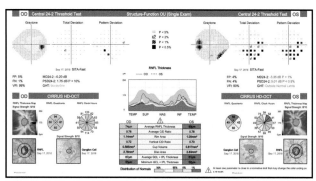

Figure 8-1B. The visual field (Humphrey Field Analyzer SITA Fast [Zeiss]) shows a few points flagged inferior. The left eye also has a large optic disc (2.83 mm²) with an average RNFL of 60 μm. The rim is thin superiorly, as seen by the Temporal Superior Nasal Inferior Temporal curve with a corresponding inferior visual field defect. Given the extent of damage, especially in OS, this requires a 40% target IOP reduction that will probably require, at a minimum, 2 medications to bring it to this level.

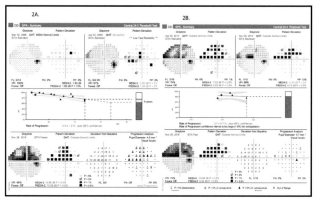

Figure 8-2. (A) The Guided Progression Analysis visual fields are seen for this individual with primary open-angle glaucoma. Progression was confirmed in 2014 and a medication (Simbrinza [brimonidine/brinzolamide ophthalmic]) added to the therapeutic regimen (latanoprost). IOP received to low teens and the Guided Progression Analysis needed to be modified, as seen in B. (B) The fields are seen to be stable with little change between 2014 and 2018.

modifications to therapy must be considered. Physicians may consider changing the agent within the same class, adding a different class of medication, or performing laser/incisional surgery (depending upon the degree of damage present). If the tests are stable, the patient is continued on their present therapy with the testing sequence modified. However, individuals may progress at any time; if change is discovered, the testing interval must be modified with progression confirmed with follow-up testing.

WHEN TO ADVANCE TREATMENT

As with beginning treatment, at all follow-up visits, the patient is questioned about how often they use their drops, problems with eye drop instillation, side effects, and trouble with cost. The physician must help the patient troubleshoot the problems associated with the use of long-term medical therapy.

The minimum IOP reduction considered satisfactory is 15%. However, when the baseline IOP is in the lower range, it may be difficult to get even a small reduction. When the IOP reduces but does not reach target level, the clinician must decide if further therapy is warranted. If further therapy is needed, the initial PGA can be switched to a different one in the same class, or a medication from a different class can be added. If a medication is added, it is preferable to choose a medication with a complementary mechanism of action, also keeping the patient's needs in mind. Some clinicians will add a fixed-combination agent to a PGA to lower IOP. However, while fixed-combination agents have the advantage of usually providing significant IOP lowering, there is concern that if there are side effects or a lack of efficacy, it may not be clear which medication is causing the problem. For this reason, many clinicians still begin medications separately.

CONCLUSION

Glaucoma is a serious sight-threatening condition that requires lifelong monitoring and treatment. It is important to educate patients about the nature of this disease, as well as the risks and benefits of treatment. Despite advancements in procedural treatment modalities to control IOP, medical therapy still remains the first-line treatment for most patients. Though sometimes affected by issues of cost and adherence, medical treatment of glaucoma is a highly successful yet conservative way to keep the disease at bay.

REFERENCES

1. Alm A, Stjernschantz J, Scandinavian Latanoprost Study Group. Effects on intraocular pressure and side effects of 0.005% latanoprost applied once daily, evening and morning. A comparison with timolol. *Ophthalmology*. 1995;102(12):1743-1752.
2. Camras CB, Alm A, Watson P, Stjernschantz J, Latanoprost Study Group. Latanoprost, a prostaglandin analog for glaucoma therapy. Efficacy and safety after 1 year of treatment in 198 patients. *Ophthalmology*. 1996;103(11):1916-1924.

3. Kraushar MF. Miotics and retinal detachment. *Arch Ophthalmol.* 1991;109(12):1659.

4. Medeiros FA, Martin KR, Peace J, et al. Comparison of latanoprostene bunod 0.024% and timolol maleate 0.5% in open-angle glaucoma or ocular hypertension. The Lunar study. *Am J Ophthalmol.* 2016;168:250-259.

5. Weinreb RN, Liebmann JM, Martin KR, Kaufman PL, Vittitow JL. Latanoprostene bunod 0.024% in subjects with open-angle glaucoma or ocular hypertension: pooled phase-3 study findings. *J Glaucoma.* 2018;27(1):7-15.

6. Weinreb RN, Ong T, Scassellati Sforzolini B, et al. A randomized controlled comparison of latanoprostene bunod and latanoprost 0.005% in the treatment of ocular hypertensive and open angle glaucoma: the Voyager Study. *Br J Ophthalmol.* 2015;99(6):738-745.

7. Zimmerman TJ, Kaufman HE. Timolol. A beta-adrenergic blocking agent for the treatment of glaucoma. *Arch Ophthalmol.* 1977;95(4):601-604.

8. Liu JH, Kripke DF, Weinreb RN. Comparison of the nocturnal effects of once daily timolol and latanoprost on intraocular pressure. *Am J Ophthalmol.* 2004;138(3):389-395.

9. Boger WP 3rd. Short-term escape and long-term drift. The dissipation effects of beta adrenergic blocking agents. *Surv Ophthalmol.* 1983;28(Suppl):235-242. Review.

10. Wilensky JT. The role of brimonidine in the treatment of open-angle glaucoma. *Surv Ophthalmol.* 1996;41(Suppl 1):S3-S7. Review.

11. Liu JH, Medeiros FA, Slight JR, Weinreb RN. Diurnal and nocturnal effects of brimonidine monotherapy on intraocular pressure. *Ophthalmology.* 2010;117(11):2075-2079.

12. Bietti G, Virno M, Pecori-Giraldi J. Acetazolamide, metabolic acidosis and intraocular pressure. *Am J Ophthalmol.* 1975;80(3 Pt 1):360-369.

13. MK-507 Clinical Study Group. Long-term glaucoma treatment with MK-507, Dorzolamide. a topical carbonic anhydrase inhibitor. *J Glaucoma.* 1995;4(1):6-10.

14. Podos SM, Serle JB. Topically active carbonic-anhydrase inhibitors for glaucoma. *Arch Ophthalmol.* 1991;109(1):38-40.

15. Liu JH, Medeiros FA, Slight JR, Weinreb RN. Comparing diurnal and nocturnal effects of brinzolamide and timolol on intraocular pressure in patients receiving latanoprost monotherapy. *Ophthalmology.* 2009;116(3):449-454.

16. Kanski JJ. Miotics. *Br J Ophthalmol.* 1968;52(12):936-937.

17. Ren R, Li G, Le TD, et al. Netarsudil increases outflow facility in human eyes through muliptle mechanisms. *Invest Ophthalmol Vis Sci.* 2016;57(14):6197-6209.

18. Serle JB, Katz LJ, McLaurin E, et al. Two phase 3 clinical trials comparing the safety and efficacy of netarsudil to timolol in patients with elevated intracoula presure. Rho kinase elevated IOP treatment trial 1 and 2 (Rocket-1 and Rocket-2) study groups. *Am J Ophthalmol.* 2018;186:116-127.

19. Tanna AP, Johnson M. Rho kinase inhibitors as a novel treatment for open angle glaucoma and ocular hypertension. *Ophthalmology.* 2018;125(11):1741-1756.

20. European Glaucoma Society. Terminology and guidelines for glaucoma. Chapter 3: treatment principles and options. *Br J Ophthalmol.* 2017;101(6):130-195.

21. Realini T. Frequency of asymmetric intraocular pressure fluctuations among patients with and without glaucoma. *Ophthalmology.* 2002;109(7):1367-1371.

22. Realini T, Fechtner RD, Atreides SP, Gollance S. The uniocular drug trial and second-eye response to glaucoma medications. *Ophthalmology.* 2004;111(3):421-426.

23. Realini T, Vickers WR. Symmetry of fellow-eye intraocular pressure responses to topical glaucoma medications. *Ophthalmology.* 2005;112(4):599-602.

24. Realini T, Weinreb RN, Wisniewski SR. Diurnal intraocular-pressure patterns are not repeatable in the short-term in healthy individuals. *Ophthalmology.* 2010;117(4):1700-1704.

25. Realini TD. A prospective, randomized, investigator-masked evaluation of the monocular trial in ocular hypertension or open-angle glaucoma. *Ophthalmology.* 2009;116(7):1237-1242.

26. Realini T. Assessing the effectiveness of intraocular pressure lowering therapy. *Ophthalmology.* 2010;117(11):2045-2046.

27. Crabb DP, Garway-Heath DF. Intervals between visual fields when monitoring the glaucomatous patient. Wait-and see-approach. *Invest Ophthalmol Vis Sci.* 2012;53(6):2770-2776.

28. Chauhan BC, Garway-Heath DF, Goni FJ, et al. Practical recommendations for measuring rates of visual field change in glaucoma. *Br J Ophthalmol.* 2008;92(4):569-573.

29. Crabb DP, Russell RA, Malik R, et al. Frequency of visual field testing when monitoring patients newly diagnosed with glaucoma: mixed methods and modelling. *Health Serv Deliv Res.* 2014;2(27):1-102.

30. Filippopoulos T, Paula JS, Torun N, et al. Periorbital changes associated with bimatoprost. *Ophthalmic Plast Reconstr Surg.* 2008;24(4):302-307.

9

Microinvasive Glaucoma Surgery
Trabecular Bypass/Ablation Procedures

Iqbal "Ike" K. Ahmed, MD
and Anna T. Do, MD

INTRODUCTION

Direct gonioscopy is a critical skill one must master in order to succeed in performing most microinvasive glaucoma surgery procedures. Direct gonioscopy is performed with the patient in a supine position with their head turned 30 degrees away from the surgeon. The microscope is tilted 30 to 45 degrees away from the surgeon, with the oculars adjusted upward for surgeon comfort. Optimal angle visualization occurs when the degree of microscope tilt matches the degree of patient head turn. The goal is to view the angle structures as if the surgeon is facing a straight wall with the iris parallel to the injector of the device being implanted/ utilized. The usual mistake is that the head and/or microscope is not rotated enough. Using a direct gonioscopy lens (Koeppe, Hoskins-Barkan, Swan-Jacob, or Richardson lens) along with a coupling agent (most commonly a viscoelastic), the lens is gently

Panarelli JF, ed.
The Pocket Guide to Glaucoma (pp 141-150).
© 2022 Taylor & Francis Group.

placed on the ocular surface to view an upright, direct image of the angle. A modified Swan Jacobs lens is most commonly used, as it is easy to manipulate and provides an optimal view of the angle.

SCHLEMM'S CANAL–BASED MICROSTENTS

There are 3 US Food and Drug Administration (FDA)–approved microstents for ab interno insertion into Schlemm's canal (SC): iStent (Glaukos Corp), iStent inject (Glaukos Corp), and the Hydrus Microstent (Ivantis Inc). Each of these microstents comes in a preloaded inserter and is designed to be injected via an ab interno approach into SC to facilitate aqueous egress from the anterior chamber to the distal collector channel system.

iStent

The first-generation iStent is composed of nonferromagnetic titanium with heparin coating, and measures 1.0 mm in length with a 120 μm snorkel. It is FDA-approved for placement in conjunction with cataract surgery in patients with mild-to-moderate open-angle glaucoma (OAG). Samuelson et al randomized 240 eyes to cataract surgery plus iStent or cataract surgery alone and found a 22% difference in the proportion of patients in the iStent group with an unmedicated intraocular pressure (IOP) ≤ 21 mm Hg compared to the control group at 12 months (72% vs 50%, $P < .001$).[1] In addition, there was a significant difference in the proportion of patients who achieved at least a 20% IOP decrease without ocular hypotensive medication (66% cataract plus iStent vs 48% cataract alone). There were no vision-threatening complications observed during the study period. Reported iStent-related complications include hyphema (0% to 70%), stent malposition (2.6% to 3%), and stent obstruction (4% to 30%).

Placement of this device begins with piercing the trabecular meshwork (TM) followed by relaxing the hand (imagine slightly pulling the TM toward you) then pivoting within the temporal wound in order to gently slide the device into the canal.

Movement of the eye suggests that the iStent is hitting the back wall of SC. The most common mistake is pushing the device into the angle rather than sliding behind the TM, just anterior to the outer wall of SC. Any loss of visualization due to bleeding should be dealt with immediately. Remember to push the reflux of blood away from the area of interest by injecting viscoelastic, similar to how a leaf blower can be used to push debris to the side. The surgeon should be cognizant of where they intend to make the next attempt and avoid displacing blood reflux into that region.

iStent Inject

The second-generation iStent inject was approved by the FDA in 2018 for use in conjunction with cataract surgery. The iStent inject is a titanium device coated in heparin and is 360 μm in length, with a maximal width of 230 μm. It is directly implanted into SC instead of requiring cannulation, as with the first-generation iStent. The handpiece comes preloaded with 2 microstents. The implanted head resides in SC and contains 4 side-flow orifices, and the flange resides in the anterior chamber with an inlet orifice.[2] The US Investigational Device Exemption pivotal trial randomized patients with mild-to-moderate glaucoma to iStent plus cataract surgery (n = 387) or cataract surgery alone (n = 118). The investigators found the iStent inject group achieved a statistically significant reduction in unmedicated IOP, with 75.3% of iStent inject plus cataract surgery cohort achieving a 20% reduction in IOP compared to 61.9% in the cataract-only cohort at 24 months. The most common postoperative issues with the iStent inject were inability to visualize both stents (13%),[3] stent obstruction (1% to 3%),[3] and IOP spike (1%).

The device is placed differently than the first-generation iStent. The trocar is used to pierce the TM perpendicularly to cause a slight dimpling of the TM, then inject the stent by pressing the injector button on the handpiece (Figure 9-1). Applying too much force will result in a misfire and the stent may not deploy. Not having enough pressure to create a dimple may lead to superficial deployment. Once the TM is punctured by the trocar, the

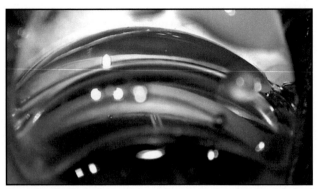

Figure 9-1. iStent inject being deployed. Note positioning of trochar at the level of the TM. Gentle forward bias is required as the stent is being delivered.

surgeon must then ensure that the trocar is centered within the shaft of the injector. This ensures neutral forces are not biased to one direction over the others. The most common error is to have a slight bend in the trocar that equates to potential energy that will manifest as a side flick once the injector button is pushed. Stents are usually either misfired and/or the trocar can be bent rendering the injector damaged for deploying stents.

Hydrus Microstent

The Hydrus Microstent was approved by the FDA in 2018 for implantation with cataract surgery. The device is a preloaded flexible, 8 mm, metal (nitinol), curved scaffold with windows that stent open SC. The device spans 90 degrees of the patient's canal to increase outflow through the conventional pathway. The HORIZON study randomized 369 eyes to cataract surgery with Hydrus Microstent and 187 eyes to cataract surgery alone and followed the patients for 24 months.[4] The results showed that the unmedicated IOP was reduced by ≥ 20% in 77.3% of the Hydrus Microstent group compared to 57.8% of the no microstent group eyes (difference = 19.5%, 95% confidence interval 11.2% to 27.8%, $P < .001$). In addition, the number of medications was reduced by 1.4 in the Hydrus Microstent group compared to 1.0 in the cataract surgery-alone group ($P < .001$). The COMPARE trial, which randomized eyes to receive Hydrus Microstent as a standalone treatment in phakic patients or 2 iStents, found that the Hydrus outperformed 2 iStents in regards to reducing medication requirement at 12 months (46.6% of Hydrus patients were medication-free compared to 24% of iStent patients).[5]

The most common complication after Hydrus Microstent implantation is peripheral anterior synechiae (PAS) formation (18% of patients with focal 1 to 2 mm PAS in the Hydrus II study).[6] Other potential postoperative complications include intraoperative or postoperative hyphema,[4] macular edema (2%),[6] and transient IOP spike (2% to 6.5%).[6,7] If iris adhesions to the implant develop and obstruct flow, argon laser can be used to attempt to relieve microstent obstruction.

The technique with Hydrus is different than TM stenting with an iStent. An incision must be made just lateral (right-handed surgeons must be 1 to 2 clock hours to the right) to the traditional temporal incision. The injector must pierce the TM as the slider is advanced forward, pressure must be released (relax the hand and avoid indenting the TM) in order to safely deploy the device. If there is significant resistance, the device may need to be withdrawn and inserted into another clock hour. This can either be achieved going the opposite direction or positioning the scope from temporal to superior to aim for the inferior angle. Remember to make another incision just lateral to what would be directly in line with the intended area of placement.

Trabecular Ablative Procedures

Kahook Dual Blade

The Kahook Dual Blade (KDB; New World Medical) is a single-use, disposable device designed to excise a portion of the TM. The device has a sharp edge that allows entry into the TM, while 2 sharp goniotomy blades excise a strip of TM. The KDB allows for complete removal of the TM (in contrast to microvitreoretinal blade goniotomy and the gonioscopy-assisted transluminal trabeculotomy) and does not cause thermal injury to nearby tissue (in contrast to the trabectome).[8] The KDB goniotomy is approved as a standalone procedure or in combination with cataract surgery. While this device is most often used in patients with primary OAG, it may be particularly useful in patients with secondary OAGs (pseudoexfoliative and pigmentary glaucoma), as the outflow obstruction is primarily at the level of the TM in these conditions. There has also been reported success with KDB goniotomy in cases of congenital, steroid-induced, and uveitic glaucomas.[9]

Intraoperative reflux of blood, if severe, may obscure the surgeon's view; this may be managed with judicious addition of viscoelastic into the anterior chamber to tapenade the bleeding. The most common postoperative adverse events after KDB goniotomy include hyphema (34.9%), pain/irritation (7.7%), and IOP spike > 10 mm Hg (3.8% to 12.6%).[10] These complications tend to be self-limited and transient.

As with other microinvasive glaucoma surgery devices, the KDB is inserted through a clear corneal wound, and direct visualization of the angle is required to perform the procedure. There are various ways to perform this procedure, but the general principles are the same. The surgeon inserts the device and engages the TM 2 to 3 clock hours to the right (or left) of center. The canal is entered with the sharp edge of the blade (may be helpful to direct the distal tip of the KDB up 10 degrees toward Schwalbe's line). The heel of the KDB is then rested back on the anterior wall of the canal and advanced from right to left (Figure 9-2). The TM should rise over the ramp as parallel incisions are made with the dual blade. The surgeon should advance the blade smoothly for several clock hours and then stop. The same exact procedure is performed from the opposite direction, and the strip of amputated TM is joined and removed. The viscoelastic is then removed, and the anterior chamber is inflated to an IOP between 20 to 30 mm Hg. Higher pressure and closure of wounds (recommend suturing main wound) helps prevent bleeding and hyphema formation in the early postoperative period.

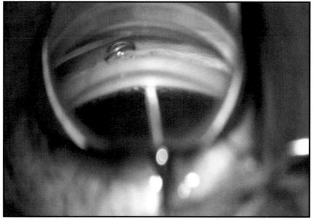

Figure 9-2. KDB engaging the TM just off-center. The KDB will be advanced from right to left for several clock hours, and the same approach will be taken from the opposite side to join the cut segments at the midpoint.

Trabectome

The trabectome is a surgical instrument that is used for electroablative ab interno trabeculectomy (Neomedix Corp). The instrument consists of a bipolar 550 kHz electrode with adjustable power settings (typically 0.8 to 1.0 W) to ablate the TM. The handpiece includes an 18.5-gauge infusion sleeve and a 25-gauge ablation tip that is powered by a footplate. Viscoelastic is not used to avoid optical interfaces and trapping of ablation bubbles. The infusion helps to maintain the chamber and aides in aspiration of the ablated tissue debris. Through a uniplanar 1.6 mm clear corneal incision, up to 180 degrees of the TM can be ablated using a forehand and backhand technique. It was approved by the FDA in 2004 for the treatment of glaucoma and may be used in phakic, pseudophakic, or aphakic eyes—as long as the gonioscopic view of the angle is clear. Narrow angles have been considered a relative contraindication due to the more difficult viewing of the angle, and higher risk for peripheral anterior synechiae/fibrosis of the angle.

Postoperatively, surgeons may prefer to prescribe pilocarpine 1% to 2% for the first 8 postoperative weeks to keep the iris flat and away from the angle. Complications from trabectome include transient hyphema (almost 100% of cases), PAS formation (24%),[11] and transient IOP spike > 10 mm Hg (4% to 10%). Less common adverse effects include wrong site ablation causing damage to the ciliary body instead of the TM and cyclodialysis cleft.

The most crucial step to the trabectome procedure is setting up the device. Surgeons should familiarize themselves with the handpiece and electrocautery unit and understand the sequence of steps that need to be followed to correctly set up the device. Once the unit is ready, the protective cap should be removed by the surgeon to make sure that the delicate end of the handpiece is not damaged. Gentle pressure is applied to the posterior lip of the wound and the device is inserted across the eye. By raising the bottle height, the anterior chamber can be maintained through the infusion line, just as in traditional phacoemulsification cases. The goniolens is then placed on the eye, and the area of targeted ablation is engaged. By depressing the footswitch all the way down, the electrosurgical function is activated, and treatment can commence. Ablation is performed in 1 direction for several clock hours. Resistance or movement of the eye in the direction of the TM ablation may indicate incorrect positioning and the tip may be engaged in the inner wall of SC. To avoid this issue, the surgeon should pull back slightly while advancing to adjust for the curvature of the eye. The handpiece is then rotated 180 degrees, and treatment is completed in the opposite direction (Figure 9-3). Typical treatment is 90 to 120 degrees of the nasal angle.

CONCLUSION

Trabecular bypass microstents and trabecular ablative procedures can be safe and effective options for patients with mild-to-moderate OAG undergoing cataract surgery, but may also offer IOP-lowering options as a standalone treatment. Complications such as hyphema, stent malposition/obstruction, and IOP spikes may occur at low but discernable rates.

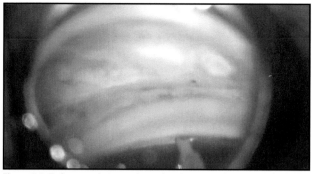

Figure 9-3. Trabectome being performed in the reverse direction. Note the difference in angle pigmentation. To the left, the TM has been ablated and a white band is seen in the location of the cleft.

REFERENCES

1. Samuelson TW, Katz LJ, Wells JM, et al. Randomized evaluation of the trabecular micro-bypass stent with phacoemulsification in patients with glaucoma and cataract. *Ophthalmology.* 2011;118:459-467.
2. Voskanyan L, García-Feijoó J, Belda JI, et al. Prospective, unmasked evaluation of the iStent inject system for open-angle glaucoma: synergy trial. *Adv Ther.* 2014;31:189-201.
3. Klamann MKJ, Gonnermann J, Pahlitzsch M, et al. iStent inject in phakic open angle glaucoma. *Graefes Arch Clin Exp Ophthalmol.* 2015;253:941-947.
4. Samuelson TW, Chang DF, Marquis R, et al. A Schlemm canal microstent for intraocular pressure reduction in primary open-angle glaucoma and cataract: the HORIZON study. *Ophthalmology.* 2019;126:29-37.
5. Chang DF. COMPARE Trial. Prospective, multicenter, randomized comparison of Hydrus versus two iStents for standalone treatment of OAG. Presented at: American Society of Cataract and Refractive Surgery annual meeting; April 13-17, 2018; Washington.
6. Pfeiffer N, Garcia-Feijoo J, Martinez-de-la-Casa JM, et al. A randomized trial of a Schlemm's canal microstent with phacoemulsification for reducing intraocular pressure in open-angle glaucoma. *Ophthalmology.* 2015;122:1283-1293.
7. Fea AM, Ahmed IK, Lavia C, et al. Hydrus microstent compared to selective laser trabeculoplasty in primary open angle glaucoma: one year results. *Clin Experiment Ophthalmol.* 2017;45:120-127.

8. Seibold LK, Soohoo JR, Ammar DA, Kahook MY. Preclinical investigation of ab interno trabeculectomy using a novel dual-blade device. *Am J Ophthalmol*. 2013;155:524-529.e2.

9. Khouri AS, Wong SH. Ab interno trabeculectomy with a dual blade: surgical technique for childhood glaucoma. *J Glaucoma*. 2017;26:749-751.

10. Dorairaj SK, Kahook MY, Williamson BK, et al. A multicenter retrospective comparison of goniotomy versus trabecular bypass device implantation in glaucoma patients undergoing cataract extraction. *Clin Ophthalmol*. 2018;12:791-797.

11. Minckler DS, Baerveldt G, Alfaro MR, Francis BA. Clinical results with the trabectome for treatment of open-angle glaucoma. *Ophthalmology*. 2005;112:962-967.

10

Canal-Based Glaucoma Surgery

*Jonathan B. Lin, MD, PhD
and Arsham Sheybani, MD*

INTRODUCTION

One subcategory of microinvasive glaucoma surgery (MIGS) includes canal-based surgeries. In contrast with traditional subconjunctival filtration approaches, which generate a new route of aqueous humor outflow, canal-based surgery augments existing outflow pathways to reduce intraocular pressure (IOP). The aim of this chapter is to highlight 3 canal-based glaucoma surgeries: ab interno canaloplasty (ABiC), gonioscopy-assisted transluminal trabeculotomy (GATT), and the OMNI Glaucoma Treatment System (Sight Sciences, Inc). Given their balance of safety and efficacy, these surgical approaches show promise for patients who do not need IOPs below episcleral venous pressure.

Panarelli JF, ed.
151   *The Pocket Guide to Glaucoma* (pp 151-157).
© 2022 Taylor & Francis Group.

AB INTERNO CANALOPLASTY

Overview

ABiC is a surgical technique that involves circumferential catheterization of Schlemm's canal (SC) with an illuminated microcatheter (iTrack [Nova Eye Medical]) to perform viscodilation of the outflow system. SC is catheterized through a side-port incision in the cornea under direct gonioscopic visualization. It is thought that ABiC achieves IOP reduction by dilating a collapsed SC, stretching compressed trabecular meshwork (TM), and clearing mechanical obstruction in the collector channel system. ABiC restores the physiologic outflow pathway rather than creating a new outflow tract in the sclera. This approach does not require conjunctival or scleral dissection, nor does it require placement of an intraluminal tensioning suture.

Evidence

In a study sponsored by Ellex, the manufacturer of the patented microcatheter, ABiC was found to be effective at reducing both IOP and the need for IOP-lowering medication after 1 year of follow-up.[1] This retrospective, single-center case series tracked outcomes for 75 eyes of 68 primary open-angle glaucoma (POAG) patients following ABiC, performed either as a standalone procedure or in conjunction with cataract extraction. On average, ABiC reduced IOP from 20.4 mm Hg to 13.3 mm Hg. Moreover, POAG patients who underwent ABiC had a significant reduction in the average number of glaucoma medications (from 2.8 to 1.1), with 40% of eyes medication-free. Both the IOP reduction and the reduction in medications were similar in the ABiC-alone group and the ABiC/Phaco group. Another retrospective case series of 36 eyes of 28 POAG patients had similar findings at 1-year follow-up, although these authors did not find a significant reduction in the number of IOP-lowering medications.[2] Given its relative infancy, long-term studies are necessary to assess the durability of ABiC beyond 1 year.

Advantages and Disadvantages

Unlike other glaucoma surgeries, ABiC spares the sclera and requires minimal conjunctival manipulation. It can be performed concurrently with cataract extraction and adds minimal additional risk in the hands of an experienced surgeon. ABiC does not preclude future, more invasive glaucoma surgery. Technical challenges associated with ABiC can lead to intraoperative complications, including difficulty in cannulating SC, Descemet membrane detachment, or improper microcatheter passage. Although adverse events are rare, there have been reports of hyphema, cataract formation, IOP spikes, and hypotony following ABiC. Since these complications rarely lead to long-term visual consequences, ABiC is considered a low-risk procedure.

GONIOSCOPY-ASSISTED TRANSLUMINAL TRABECULOTOMY

Overview

Trabeculotomy is an approach for reducing IOP based on the principle that the TM generates a significant proportion of the resistance to aqueous humor outflow.[3] It is believed that opening up the TM enhances outflow and thereby decreases IOP. Though trabeculotomy has traditionally been performed via an ab externo approach, it can now be performed via an ab interno approach under direct gonioscopic visualization (ie, GATT). GATT involves passing a suture—or illuminated microcatheter—into the anterior chamber through a side-port incision in the cornea and then passed circumferentially around SC. Once the canal is threaded 360 degrees, the loop is pulled into the anterior chamber to create a trabecular shelf. Like ABiC, GATT opens up the physiologic outflow pathway rather than generating a new pathway for aqueous humor flow. Although complete 360-degree canalization cannot always be achieved depending on the patient's anatomy, partial trabeculotomy should also theoretically yield an IOP-lowering benefit.

Evidence

GATT was first described in 2014 in a retrospective case series of 85 patients.[4] At 1 year, the 57 POAG patients who underwent GATT had an average IOP reduction of 11.1 mm Hg and an average reduction in medications of 1.1. Only 9% of the patients in this case series were considered GATT failures at 1 year (required additional glaucoma surgery). Patients with secondary OAG who underwent GATT also achieved similar IOP reductions and similar reductions in medications. Though GATT appears to be most suitable for patients with OAG, there have been reports suggesting its benefit in pediatric patients with congenital/juvenile glaucoma as well as in adults with refractory glaucoma.[5,6]

Advantages and Disadvantages

Like ABiC, GATT requires similar incisions for access and can also be performed concurrently with cataract extraction. Since it does not involve scleral or conjunctival manipulation, it also does not preclude future, more invasive glaucoma surgery. Another advantage of GATT is that it is cost-effective, as it can be performed with only a suture, thermal cautery, viscoelastic, and microforceps (some surgeons always prefer to use the illuminated microcatheter, which is more costly). Although the technical challenges of GATT are similar to ABiC, one potential disadvantage that is unique is the increased likelihood of postoperative hyphema, especially in patients who are unable to stop anticoagulation or are, for some other reason, prone to bleeding. Although this can resolve on its own, it sometimes requires anterior chamber washout. Nonetheless, this complication rarely leads to long-term visual consequences.

OMNI GLAUCOMA TREATMENT SYSTEM

Overview

The OMNI Glaucoma Treatment System combines both the previous strategies. Like both ABiC and GATT, circumferential catheterization of SC is achieved through a minimally invasive approach. The OMNI system can thereafter be used for both transluminal viscodilation and subsequent unroofing of the TM. In essence, the OMNI system combines the strategies of GATT with ABiC in a single handheld device, although 1 potential limitation is that the device may not pressurize the collector system as high as ABiC does.

Evidence

A prospective, multicenter, single-arm study of 137 patients to evaluate the safety and efficacy of the OMNI system in conjunction with cataract extraction recently reported favorable interim results at the 6-month time point.[7] Final 1-year data are not yet available.

Advantages and Disadvantages

The combination of trabeculotomy and viscocanaloplasty might theoretically yield improved IOP reduction compared to either intervention-alone with a similar profile of peri- and postoperative complications. Nonetheless, future studies are necessary to determine whether this remains true in real-world practice.

Conclusion

One overarching advantage of canal-based approaches is that they are minimally invasive and thus do not preclude future trabeculectomy or other MIGS approaches, if additional IOP reduction is necessary. Since these procedures have favorable safety profiles, it is reasonable to pursue these canal-based approaches early in the disease course in patients who require moderate IOP reduction. Although long-term studies examining the durability of these approaches are not available, these canal-based approaches show considerable promise.

One limitation of the existing evidence for canal-based approaches is that they are mainly single-arm case series. Future studies are needed to determine how these canal-based approaches compare to other surgical interventions, including other canal-based approaches and other MIGS approaches altogether. These studies would provide much needed information about how these interventions differ from one another and, thereby, help guide treatment approaches. It would be of further interest to determine whether there are certain patient or disease characteristics that predict favorable response to a particular MIGS approach, as these would provide helpful guidance of determining the optimal treatment pathway for each individual patient.

Acknowledgments

Jonathan B. Lin was supported by the National Institutes of Health grants T32 GM07200, UL1 TR002345, and TL1 TR002344. Arsham Sheybani receives consulting fees from Allergan and Katena.

REFERENCES

1. Gallardo MJ, Supnet RA, Ahmed IK. Viscodilation of Schlemm's canal for the reduction of IOP via an ab-interno approach. *Clin Ophthalmol.* 2018;12:2149-2155.

2. Davids AM, Pahlitzsch M, Boeker A, et al. Ab interno canaloplasty (ABiC)—12-month results of a new minimally invasive glaucoma surgery (MIGS). *Graefes Arch Clin Exp Ophthalmol.* 2019;257(9):1947-1953.

3. Rosenquist R, Epstein D, Melamed S, Johnson M, Grant WM. Outflow resistance of enucleated human eyes at two different perfusion pressures and different extents of trabeculotomy. *Curr Eye Res.* 1989;8(12):1233-1240.

4. Grover DS, Godfrey DG, Smith O, et al. Gonioscopy-assisted transluminal trabeculotomy, ab interno trabeculotomy: technique report and preliminary results. *Ophthalmology.* 2014;121(4):855-861.

5. Grover DS, Smith O, Fellman RL, et al. Gonioscopy assisted transluminal trabeculotomy: an ab interno circumferential trabeculotomy for the treatment of primary congenital glaucoma and juvenile open angle glaucoma. *Br J Ophthalmol.* 2015;99(8):1092-1096.

6. Grover DS, Godfrey DG, Smith O, et al. Outcomes of gonioscopy-assisted transluminal trabeculotomy (GATT) in eyes with prior incisional glaucoma surgery. *J Glaucoma.* 2017;26(1):41-45.

7. Gallardo MJ, Sarkisian SR Jr, Vold SD, et al. Canaloplasty and trabeculotomy combined with phacoemulsification in open-angle glaucoma: interim results from the GEMINI study. *Clin Ophthalmol.* 2021;15:481-489.

11

Microinvasive Glaucoma Surgery
Suprachoroidal Drainage Devices

Jing Wang, MD

INTRODUCTION

The suprachoroidal space is a potential space that offers an outflow pathway with significant intraocular pressure (IOP)–lowering capacity. Under normal physiological conditions, the suprachoroidal or the uveoscleral outflow pathway is estimated to account for 10% to 20% of human aqueous outflow.[1,2] In contrast to that of conventional trabecular outflow, which is IOP-dependent, uveoscleral outflow is IOP-independent. As a result of the high oncotic pressure in the uveal choroidal vessels, the suprachoroidal space has a lower pressure than the anterior chamber; this negative pressure facilitates the outflow of aqueous into the suprachoroidal space.[3] Aqueous accesses the space by permeating through ciliary muscle, the principal site of resistance in the pathway. Attempts have been made to harness the suprachoroidal pathway because of its impressive potential IOP-lowering effect without bleb formation, thereby avoiding complications such as dysesthesia and blebitis.

Panarelli JF, ed. *The Pocket Guide to Glaucoma* (pp 159-171). © 2022 Taylor & Francis Group.

There are numerous reasons to use a device to utilize the suprachoroidal pathway. First, the IOP-lowering capacity of the trabecular meshwork (TM) or Schlemm's canal–targeting devices or procedures is limited by episcleral venous pressure, whereas suprachoroidal procedures are not. Second, patients with glaucoma and elevated IOP have reduced trabecular outflow facility, so one could argue that enhancing suprachoroidal outflow would be more effective than enhancing the already dysfunctional conventional pathway (prostaglandin analogues are the most effective pharmacologic agents in reducing IOP and act on suprachoroidal outflow[4]). Third, the conventional TM pathway ultimately drains aqueous into the episcleral vessels, which are dependent on the state of the ocular surface. In patients with an inflamed ocular surface, due to toxicity or previous failed filtering surgery, enhancing the TM pathway may not be very effective. In contrast, the suprachoroidal pathway is completely independent of the ocular surface.[5]

The impressive IOP-lowering effect of the suprachoroidal pathway is illustrated by the profound hypotony that results from a traumatic cyclodialysis cleft—where detachment of ciliary muscle from scleral spur eliminates resistance to uveoscleral outflow. Iatrogenic cyclodialysis clefts have been attempted in the past, to reduce IOP as a treatment for glaucoma, using a spatula. This procedure has never gained popularity due to its high complication rate and unpredictable results: a high rate of profound hypotony followed by spontaneous closure of the cleft and an acute IOP elevation with pain and vision loss.[6] Ab externo suprachoroidal devices have been developed to keep the cleft open and control the amount filtration. The Gold Micro Shunt (SOLX) was one of the first commercially available ab externo suprachoroidal devices. It is a small rectangular device with multiple microchannels controlling flow from the anterior chamber to the suprachoroidal space.[7] Manufactured from 24-karat gold to minimize the foreign body reaction, the Gold Micro Shunt was placed under a scleral flap with the anterior portion of the shunt in the anterior chamber and the posterior portion in the suprachoroidal space. The microchannels permitted aqueous flow into the suprachoroidal space.

The scleral flap was closed tightly prior to conjunctival closure to avoid subconjunctival filtration. The STARflo Glaucoma Implant (iSTAR Medical) is a flat device that is implanted and operates in a similar fashion to the Gold Micro Shunt. STARflo is made of a silicone elastomer (STAR material) instead of gold. Aquashunt (OPKO Health) is another ab externo suprachoroidal device made of polypropylene with a similar design. The surgical technique is similar for all the ab externo devices. Conjunctival and scleral flap dissection are required for placement and the devices all connect the anterior chamber to the suprachoroidal space. High-level clinical evidence of outcomes of these devices is limited. Despite the theoretical IOP-lowering capacity, the final IOPs were higher than that obtained with traditional filtering surgery and without fewer complications.[8] Both over-filtration and scarring were associated with these devices.[9] There is currently no ab externo suprachoroidal device available in the United States. The Gold Micro Shunt is still available in Europe and Canada.

Ab interno suprachoroidal devices are minimally tissue-invasive, as they avoid conjunctival and scleral dissection. They are quicker to implant and are usually implanted in conjunction with cataract surgery. Ab interno suprachoroidal devices are delivered through a clear corneal incision via a preloaded injector (Figure 11-1). The CyPass Micro-Stent (Alcon) and iStent Supra (Glaukos Corp) are 2 such devices. The CyPass Micro-Stent was US Food and Drug Administration–approved and available in the United States until its voluntary market withdrawal in August 2018.[10] The iStent Supra is CE-marked but is not yet US Food and Drug Administration–approved and is not commercially available in Europe or the United States. The company that developed STARflo is also developing an ab interno microinvasive glaucoma surgery (MIGS) suprachoroidal device, the MINIject (iSTAR Medical; Table 11-1).

Implantation of ab interno (ie, MIGS) suprachoroidal devices requires direct gonioscopic viewing. On gonioscopy, the implants are inserted between scleral spur and ciliary body band, giving access to the suprachoroidal space.

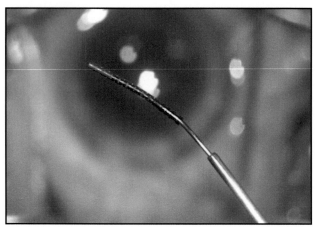

Figure 11-1. CyPass Micro-Stent threaded on to the guidewire. Three retention rings at proximal end of the tube aid in judging the correct position of the device during implantation.

CYPASS MICRO-STENT

Until recently, the CyPass Mirco-Stent was the only commercially available suprachoroidal MIGS. It is a fenestrated 6.35-mm long microstent, with external and internal diameters of 510 μm and 300 μm, respectively, and made of a biocompatible polyamide with microholes along its length to allow aqueous percolation. The anterior chamber portion of the CyPass Mirco-Stent has 3 retention rings that help in judging the correct position of the device during implantation (see Figure 11-1). The CyPass Mirco-Stent is inserted via a clear corneal incision and delivered by a guidewire (Figure 11-2). The surgical implantation technique is similar to that of trabecular bypass MIGS. Direct gonioscopic view of the angle is essential. Both the operating microscope and patient's head are rotated 30 to 40 degrees away from the surgeon. The anterior chamber is filled with viscoelastic and the angle viewed by direct gonioscopy. The guidewire directs the

Table 11-1. Summary of Different Ab Externo and Ab Interno Suprachoroidal Shunts					
AB EXTERNO SUPRACHOROIDAL DEVICES (NOT MIGS)	MATERIAL	LENGTH	WIDTH	THICKNESS	AVAILABILITY
Gold Micro-Shunt	24 karat gold	5.2 mm	3.2 mm	44 μm	Approved in Canada Investigational in United States—
STARflo	Silicone polymer	8 mm	3 to 5 mm	275 μm	CE-marked—available in Europe Unavailable in United States
Aquashunt	Polypropylene	10 mm	4 mm	750 μm	Unavailable

(continued)

Table 11-1. Summary of Different Ab Externo and Ab Interno Suprachoroidal Shunts (continued)					
AB INTERNO SUPRACHOROIDAL DEVICES (MIGS)	MATERIAL	LENGTH	INNER LUMEN	OUTER LUMEN	AVAILABILITY
CyPass Micro-Stent	Polyamide	6.35 mm	300 µm	510 µm	FDA-approved and CE-marked Unavailable due to voluntary withdrawal from market
iStent Supra	Polymer with titanium sleeve	4 mm	165 µm		CE-marked Investigational in United States

CE = Conformité Européenne (European conformity); FDA = US Food and Drug Administration; MIGS = microinvasive glaucoma surgery.

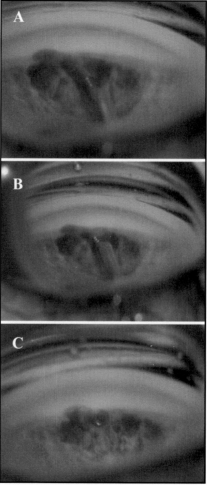

Figure 11-2. (A, B) Gonioscopic view of CyPass Micro-Stent implantation. Guidewire delivers CyPass into the suprachoroidal space. (C) View of CyPass at the angle after removal of guidewire and injector.

CyPass Micro-Stent into the suprachoroidal space at the base of scleral spur (see Figure 11-2). In contrast to TM MIGS—which are implanted between anterior and posterior TM—suprachoroidal MIGS are directed more posteriorly between scleral spur and ciliary body band. The presences of iris processes in the angle or an anterior iris insertion can hamper identification of scleral spur.

The COMPASS trial was a randomized controlled trial comparing the effect of combined cataract surgery and CyPass Mirco-Stent implantation with cataract surgery alone in 505 patients with early primary open-angle glaucoma (POAG).[11] Two years after surgery, the combined CyPass Mirco-Stent and cataract surgery group had a lower mean IOP on fewer medicines than the cataract surgery-alone group. After 2 years, 77% of combined CyPass Mirco-Stent and cataract patients achieved a 20% reduction in unmedicated IOP compared with 60% of those having cataract surgery alone. The unmedicated IOP reduction was higher in the combined CyPass Mirco-Stent and cataract surgery group than the cataract surgery-alone group: 7.4 ± 4.4 mm Hg (30%) vs 5.4 ± 3.9 mm Hg (21%). Of interest, comparable trials, involving the iStent and Hydrus, also demonstrated a sustained IOP reduction with cataract surgery alone in mild-to-moderate POAG patients. Clinicians must be careful in interpreting the IOP-lowering capacity of cataract surgery alone. All the randomized controlled trials involving either TM MIGS (iStent, Hydrus) or CyPass Mirco-Stent included early-to-moderate patients controlled on medication. The COMPASS study had a higher baseline IOP, as patients were unmedicated. Visual field progression was not an inclusion criterion in any of the above studies. Likewise, none of these studies are applicable to patients with normal-tension glaucoma, advanced POAG, POAG progressing with IOP in mid-to-low teens, or secondary glaucomas.

The DUETTE trial was a prospective series of 55 solo CyPass Mirco-Stent procedures in POAG patients with uncontrolled IOP (between 21 and 35 mm Hg) followed up for 1 year after surgery, with 35 completing 2 years of follow-up.[12,13] The authors reported effective IOP lowering with avoidance of conventional filtration surgery in 83% of patients at 1 year and 2 years of follow-up.

The IOP was reduced from 24.5 ± 2.8 mm Hg to 16.4 ± 55 mm Hg (34% IOP reduction) at 1 year and to 16.8 ± 3.9 mm Hg (31% IOP reduction) at 2 years. The CyPass Clinical Experience trial (CyCLE) was a multicenter open registry of CyPass Mirco-Stent implantations in combination with cataract surgery (n = 184), which demonstrated an average reduction in IOP of 14% (15.9 mm Hg ± 3.1 mm Hg) from baseline IOP (20.2 ± 6.0 mm Hg) with a significant reduction in glaucoma medication at 1 year.[14] The CyCLE registry reflects a cohort of patients with various types of glaucoma, including a minority with failed previous filtering surgery. Based on data from CyCLE, DUETTE trial, and the COMPASS study, the CyPass Micro-Stent can achieve an IOP reduction of between 14% to 30%.

The short-term complications associated with the CyPass Mirco-Stent include hypotony (3% to 15%), acute IOP elevation (3% to 5%), device obstruction, and migration. The hypotony associated with a CyPass Mirco-Stent is usually self-limiting. However, prolonged clinically significant hypotony can occur, especially in highly myopic eyes or in eyes with previous filtering procedures.[15]

Five years after surgery in the COMPASS XT study, there was a significantly higher rate of endothelial cell loss (ECL) in the combined CyPass Mirco-Stent and cataract group, compared with the cataract surgery-alone group (18.4% vs 7.5%). For this reason, the manufacturer voluntarily withdrew the CyPass Micro-Stent from the market in August 2018.[10] The only identifiable risk factor for ECL in the CyPass Mirco-Stent group was the number of retention rings visible on gonioscopy: The higher the number of retention rings visible, the higher the rate of ECL. The rate was 1.39% per year for eyes with no rings showing, 2.74% per year for 1 ring showing, and 6.96% per year for 2 to 3 rings showing (Figure 11-3). The reason for this increased ECL is most likely mechanical touch of a fairly rigid tube, though others have postulated increased aqueous flow close to endothelium and inflammation as potential contributors. During the 5-year COMPASS XT study, no patient with significant ECL suffered corneal decompensation or underwent corneal transplant. The current American Society

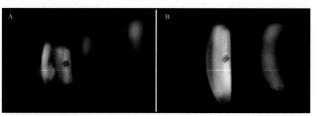

Figure 11-3. Gonioscopic view of the CyPass Micro-Stent in situ in the supraciliary space with no ring visible (A) and 1 ring visible (B).

of Cataract and Refractive Surgery's recommendation is not to remove the device, but to observe patients closely.[16] However, if ECL is confirmed and the CyPass Micro-Stent has more than one ring visible, the surgeon could consider trimming the CyPass Micro-Stent. Caution should be taken when attempting removal of the CyPass Micro-Stent, as significant fibrosis occurs in the suprachoroidal space and removal might be very traumatic.

iStent Suprachoroidal Drainage System (iStent Supra)

The iStent Supra is another suprachoroidal stent made of polyethersulfone and heparin-coated titanium with a lumen of 165 μm in diameter. The iStent Supra is not commercially available, and there are no prospective studies examining its efficacy. One published prospective study examined the combined effect of 2 trabecular iStents, 1 iStent Supra, and a topical prostaglandin in patients with advanced POAG with suboptimal IOP control.[17] All patients (n = 80) in this series had a prior failed trabeculectomy. The IOP reduced from 22.0 ± 3.1 mm Hg before implantation, to less than 13 to 14 mm Hg throughout the 4 years of follow-up. This study had a low attrition rate with 60 out of 80 patients completing 4 years of follow-up. However, the number of patients requiring further glaucoma surgery was not specified. The study was carried out in Armenia where many patients had prior filtering surgery. These results may not therefore apply to glaucoma patients in North America or Europe, where filtering surgery is reserved for patients who have failed medical treatment.

MINIJECT

The MINIject (iSTAR Medical) is a sponge-like device made of a similar material to STARflo, a porous silicone STAR material. Contrary to STARflo, which is an ab externo suprachoroidal device, MINIject is inserted into the suprachoroidal space via an ab interno approach. The MINIject is 5 mm in length with an oblong cross-section area measuring 1.1 x 0.6 mm. Two prospective noncomparative studies of 25 to 31 mild to moderate POAG patients who received MINIject as solo procedure were published (STAR I and STAR II trial).[18-20] Participants from both trials were either phakic or pseudophakic. The baseline IOP was around 24 mm Hg on 1 or more medications. At the 6-month follow-up, both series reported an average of 40% (9 mm Hg) reduction in IOP and 80% to 90% of eyes reached at least 20% IOP reduction. Cases of IOP raise were reported by both trials (STAR I, 23.1%; STAR II, 48.4%). In the STAR I trial, all cases of IOP raise were resolved by observation, discontinuation of steroid, and initiation of IOP-lowering medication; no patients required further glaucoma surgery. In the STAR II trial, the management of these cases were not reported; however, 3 patients out of 31 underwent further glaucoma surgery within 6 months of follow-up. The IOP reduction was sustained up to 24 months of follow-up in the STAR I trial.[20] Twenty-one patients completed 2 years follow-up with an average of 40.7% reduction in IOP, while 47.6% of patients were medication-free at the 24-month follow-up with IOP less than 21 mm Hg. There was a mild decrease in endothelium cell count from 2411 cells/mm^2 to 2341 cells/mm^2, reported by the STAR I trial.

Conclusion

Suprachoroidal drainage devices target a potential space where IOP lowering is not limited by episcleral venous pressure and bleb formation is not required. However, fibrosis in the suprachoroidal spaces remains an issue. The withdrawal of CyPass Micro-Stent raises the important issue of corneal endothelial health in relation to all glaucoma surgical devices. The suprachoroidal devices can potentially be an adjunct to traditional glaucoma surgery if further IOP lowering is required.[5] As of now, there are still many challenges in harnessing the suprachoroidal space.

References

1. Bill A, Phillips CI. Uveoscleral drainage of aqueous humour in human eyes. *Exp Eye Res*. 1971;12(3):275-281.

2. Brubaker RF. Measurement of uveoscleral outflow in humans. *J Glaucoma*. 2001;10(5 Suppl 1):S45-S48.

3. Emi K, Pederson JE, Toris CB. Hydrostatic pressure of the suprachoroidal space. *Invest Ophthalmol Vis Sci*. 1989;30(2):233-238.

4. Weinreb RN, Toris CB, Gabelt BT, Lindsey JD, Kaufman PL. Effects of prostaglandins on the aqueous humor outflow pathways. *Surv Ophthalmol*. 2002;47(Suppl 1):S53-S64.

5. Kerr NM, Wang J, Perucho L, Barton K. The safety and efficacy of supraciliary stenting following failed glaucoma surgery. *Am J Ophthalmol*. 2018;190:191-196.

6. Tour RL. Surgical management of glaucoma. Cyclodialysis. *Int Ophthalmol Clin*. 1963;3:151-155.

7. Melamed S, Ben Simon GJ, Goldenfeld M, Simon G. Efficacy and safety of gold micro shunt implantation to the supraciliary space in patients with glaucoma: a pilot study. *Arch Ophthalmol*. 2009;127(3):264-269.

8. Hueber A, Roters S, Jordan JF, Konen W. Retrospective analysis of the success and safety of Gold Micro Shunt Implantation in glaucoma. *BMC Ophthalmol*. 2013;13:35.

9. Oatts JT, Zhang Z, Tseng H, et al. In vitro and in vivo comparison of two suprachoroidal shunts. *Invest Ophthalmol Vis Sci*. 2013;54(8):5416-5423.

10. CyPass Micro-Stent market withdrawal. [Available from: https://www.alcon.com/content/cypass-micro-stent-market-withdrawal] Date accessed: October 11, 2018.

11. Vold S, Ahmed II, Craven ER, et al. Two-year COMPASS trial results: supraciliary microstenting with phacoemulsification in patients with open-angle glaucoma and cataracts. *Ophthalmology*. 2016;123(10):2103-2112.

12. García-Feijoo J, Rau M, Grisanti S, et al. Supraciliary micro-stent implantation for open-angle glaucoma failing topical therapy: 1-year results of a multicenter study. *Am J Ophthalmol*. 2015;159(6):1075-1081.e1.

13. García-Feijoo J, Höh H, Uzunov R, Dickerson JE. Supraciliary microstent in refractory open-angle glaucoma: two-year outcomes from the DUETTE trial. *J Ocul Pharmacol Ther*. 2018;34(7):538-542.

14. Hoeh H, Vold SD, Ahmed IK, et al. Initial clinical experience with the cypass micro-stent: safety and surgical outcomes of a novel supraciliary microstent. *J Glaucoma*. 2016;25(1):106-112.

15. Sii S, Triolo G, Barton K. Case series of hypotony maculopathy after CyPass insertion treated with intra-luminal suture occlusion. *Clin Exp Ophthalmol*. 2018;47(5):679-680.

16. ASCRS Cypass Withdrawal Task Force. Preliminary ASCRS CyPass Withdrawal Consensus Statement. Available from: https://ascrs.org/CyPass_Statement.

17. Myers JS, Masood I, Hornbeak DM, et al. Prospective evaluation of two iStent. *Adv Ther*. 2018;35(3):395-407.

18. Denis P, Hirneiß C, Reddy KP, et al. A first-in-human study of the efficacy and safety of MINIject in patients with medically uncontrolled open-angle glaucoma (STAR-I). *Ophthalmol Glaucoma*. 2019;2:290-297.

19. Garcia Feijoo J, Denis P, Hirneiß C, et al. A European study of the performance and safety of MINIject in patients with medically uncontrolled open-angle glaucoma (STAR-II). *J Glaucoma*. 2020;29(10):864-871

20. Denis P, Hirneiß C, Durr GM, et al. Two-year outcomes of the MINIject drainage system for uncontrolled glaucoma from the STAR-I first-in-human trial. *Br J Ophthalmol*. Epub ahead of print: 2020 Oct 3. doi:10.1136/ bjophthalmol-2020- 316888

12

Subconjunctival/ Sub-Tenon's Implants

Eunmee Yook, MD
and Davinder S. Grover, MD, MPH

INTRODUCTION

Glaucoma therapy centers around achieving an intraocular pressure (IOP) that prevents optic nerve atrophy and visual field loss. Initial treatment typically begins with topical pressure-lowering medications, but not all patients are able to be managed on eyedrops due to compliance, intolerance, or the severity of disease. Escalation of care involves laser procedures, incisional glaucoma surgery, or newer options, such as microinvasive glaucoma surgery (MIGS). These new minimally invasive procedures offer a reliable way of controlling IOP with a potentially lower risk of complications, such as blebitis, endophthalmitis, corneal decompensation, and vision loss. Because of this favorable side effect profile, physicians are choosing to perform MIGS on patients at earlier stages of disease.

A careful preoperative assessment, including gonioscopy and inspection of conjunctival mobility (if prior procedures have been performed), is needed to achieve success with any glaucoma

Panarelli JF, ed.
The Pocket Guide to Glaucoma (pp 173-188).
© 2022 Taylor & Francis Group.

surgical procedure. It is important to provide realistic expectations to the patient, so they understand the possibility of needing further interventions if the initial surgery is not sufficient in controlling IOP.

Currently there are several MIGS approved for the treatment of glaucoma and are divided into 3 physiologic categories: (1) increase trabecular outflow, (2) decrease aqueous inflow, and (3) subconjunctival filtration. This chapter will focus on 2 new subconjunctival filtration procedures: US Food and Drug Administration (FDA)–approved Xen Gel Stent (Allergan) and the investigational PreserFlo MicroShunt (Santen).

XEN GEL STENT

The Xen Gel Stent is a 6.0-mm stent made of porcine gelatin. Once the stent is deployed, the gelatin matrix becomes hydrated, and this allows for retention of the implant in the desired location. The internal lumen diameter measures 45 μm. The length and luminal diameter of the device create an internal resistance to limit aqueous outflow and protect against hypotony. The stent can be placed as a standalone procedure or in combination with cataract surgery and is indicated in patients with refractory open-angle glaucoma, including pseudoexfoliative and pigmentary glaucoma.

Steps to ab interno Xen:

1. A 1-mm corneal paracentesis is made in the superior temporal quadrant through which preservative-free lidocaine is injected followed by a cohesive viscoelastic.

2. A 1.8-mm keratome is used to make a corneal incision in the temporal or inferior temporal quadrant. Rotate the globe inferiorly with a second instrument and mark the conjunctiva 2.0 mm from the limbus, which will serve as the target exit point in the superior or superior-nasal quadrant.

3. Place the preloaded inserter inside the eye with the bevel up through a clear corneal incision and advance across the eye (Figure 12-1A).

4. With the lever completely pulled back on the inserter, place the 27-gauge injector needle through just slightly anterior to the trabecular meshwork. A surgical goniolens should be used to directly view the angle and guide the needle, but once location is established, the goniolens can be taken off and the eye can be stabilized with the second instrument. Make sure to engage the tip of the injector through the inner wall of the eye to ensure it remains in place after removing the gonioprism from the eye.

5. Place forward pressure to tunnel the needle through the sclera until the needle is in the subconjunctival space 2.0 mm from the limbus. Tent up the conjunctiva with the tip of the injector needle to ensure the Xen Gel Stent is deployed in the subconjunctival space (Figure 12-1B).

6. Slide the lever forward to deploy the stent and retract the needle back into the inserter. Maintain forward bias to avoid a flick with the injector that can leave the Xen long in the anterior chamber or fracture the implant. One key trick is to pause once the slider is roughly 50% advanced. At this point, the gel stent is mostly deployed, and the needle begins to retract into the injector. Let the eye return to its "ortho" position so that when the needle retracts from the wall of the inner eye, there is not torque on the globe, which can lead to a flick.

7. Remove the inserter from the eye.

8. Position can be reconfirmed with a goniolens (Figure 12-2). The ideal stent position is 1.0 mm in the anterior chamber, 2.0 mm intrascleral, and 3.0 mm in the subconjunctival space.

9. Use a blunt cannula to confirm presence of a straight, freely mobile stent in the subconjunctival space.

10. In the case of a closed conjunctival approach, the authors make a 30-gauge incision through the conjunctiva, roughly 4 to 5 mm temporal to the Xen. The Grover-Fellman (GF) microshunt spatula (Epsilon USA) is then inserted through this small incision and tunneled over to the gel stent (Figure 12-3). The Tenon's capsule that surrounds the Xen is then swept posteriorly toward the fornix with careful sweeps

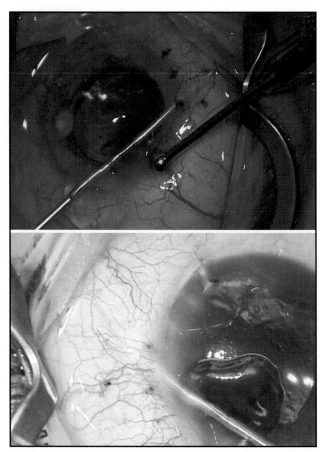

Figure 12-1. (A) Closed conjunctiva ab interno insertion of Xen Gel Stent. (B) Tenting up conjunctiva with tip of Xen inserter.

of spatula both anterior and posterior to the Xen (Figures 12-4A, 12-4B, and 12-4C). One can appreciate the Tenon's window in the operating room (Figure 12-4D) after the sweep, as well as in the clinic (Figure 12-4E).

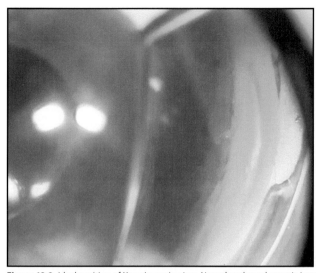

Figure 12-2. Ideal position of Xen via gonio view. Note that the gel stent is just anterior to the trabecular meshwork.

11. Once the gel stent is found to be in the ideal position, one can use the same small conjunctival incision to inject 0.1 cc of 2% lidocaine far posterior to the Xen and then use the GF micro-shunt spatula to massage the lidocaine posteriorly. Then, inject 40 to 70 mcg of mitomycin C (MMC; usually 0.15 mL of 0.4 mg/mL of MMC) far posterior to the Xen, in the area where one expects aqueous to be shunted (Figure 12-5). Massage the MMC into the focal area posterior to the Xen.

12. If a conjunctival peritomy was performed, close the fornix-based incision with a 9-0 polyglactin or nylon suture, and Step 10 cannot be performed. However, in the case of an open conjunctival approach, one can consider removing a portion of Tenon's capsule around the gel stent.

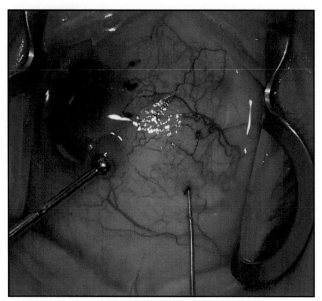

Figure 12-3. Initial entry of the GF spatula into the subconjunctival space, following uncomplicated ab interno insertion of the gel stent.

Steps to ab externo Xen with opening of conjunctiva:

1. Place a corneal traction suture at the 12:00 position.

2. Inject an aliquot of subconjunctival MMC 0.05 to 0.2 mL at a concentration between 0.1 to 0.2 mg/mL beneath the superior bulbar conjunctiva 10 mm posterior to the limbus. Alternatively, sponges soaked in the desired MMC concentration can be placed on the scleral bed for 2 to 3 minutes after Step 6. When sponges are used, the scleral bed and surrounding tissue should be rinsed with copious amounts of balanced salt solution.

3. Massage the MMC into the desired location with care to avoid letting the antimetabolite reach the limbal tissue. Rinse the surface of the eye with balanced salt solution to clear the surface of unbound MMC.

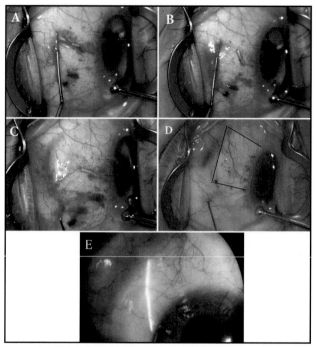

Figure 12-4. (A) Initial posterior Tenon's sweep with the GF microshunt spatula in an attempt to free the gel stent from surrounding Tenon's capsules. (B) Tenon's capsule being swept posteriorly away from the gel stent. (C) Tenon's window with gel stent free from surrounding Tenon's tissue. (D) A Tenon's window (noted by the black lines) created after a posterior Tenon's sweep. (E) Postoperative 5-month view of a patient that had a successful posterior Tenon's sweep following a gel stent.

4. Using Vannas scissors (Katena Products, Inc) and conjunctival forceps, create a fornix-based 3 mm conjunctival peritomy at the superior limbus.

5. Dissect posteriorly and laterally 3 to 4 mm adjacent to the borders of the incision.

6. Achieve hemostasis with bipolar cautery to visualize the scleral bed.

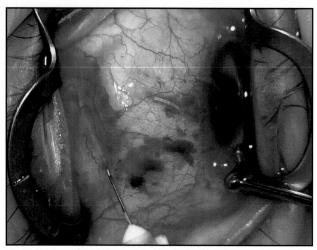

Figure 12-5. Injection of MMC into the bunched up Tenon's following a posterior Tenon's sweep with the GF microshunt spatula.

7. Stabilize the eye with 0.12 forceps and use the preloaded inserter with the needle bevel up to create a scleral tunnel starting from 2.5 mm from the limbus to the anterior chamber (Figure 12-6).

8. Slide the blue lever forward to deploy the stent and retract the needle back into the inserter.

9. Remove the inserter from the eye.

10. Position of the stent in the angle can be confirmed with a goniolens. The ideal stent position is 1.0 mm in the anterior chamber, 2.0 mm subconjunctival, and 3.0 mm in sclera (Figure 12-7).

11. Bring the conjunctiva and Tenon's flap over the implant and close at the limbus using several polyglactin or nylon sutures to create a watertight seal.

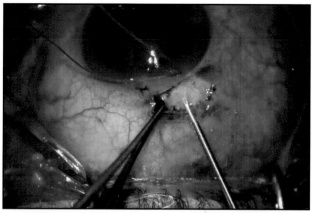

Figure 12-6. Ab externo Xen with opening of conjunctiva needle pass.

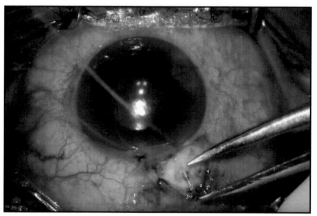

Figure 12-7. Ab externo Xen with opening of conjunctiva position of stent.

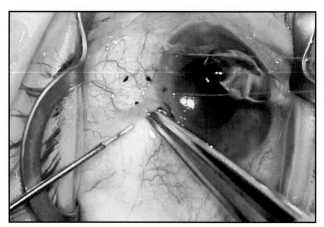

Figure 12-8. Closed conjunctiva ab externo insertion of Xen Gel Stent with pinching of conjunctiva in the superior temporal quadrant. Note that the tissue is being dragged into the inferior nasal direction.

Steps to ab externo Xen without opening conjunctiva:

1. Place a corneal traction suture at the 12 o'clock position.

2. Mark 2.5 mm posterior to the limbus. The authors have found that when one marks 2.5 mm to the limbus, by the time the injector engages the sclera for this ab externo approach, the actual scleral tunnel ends up to be around 2.0 mm.

3. Using the preloaded inserter and conjunctival forceps, pinch the superior temporal conjunctiva and drag the conjunctiva in the inferior nasal quadrant (Figure 12-8).

4. When the needle is 2.5 mm from the limbus, pass the tip of the injector needle through the conjunctiva, Tenon's capsule, and tunnel into the anterior chamber. Make sure the needle is parallel to the iris and enters the anterior chamber just at Schwalbe's line. With your nondominant hand, use the traction suture to control the globe and provide appropriate counter traction as needed (Figure 12-9).

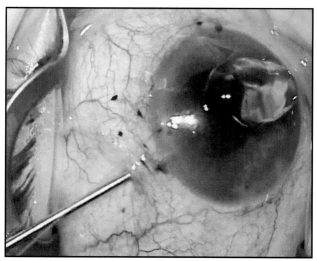

Figure 12-9. Ab externo close conjunctival pass of the gel stent. Note that the injector is entering the sclera 2 mm posterior to the limbus and the anterior bevel of the injector can be appreciated in the anterior chamber, parallel to the iris.

5. Slide the blue lever forward to deploy the stent and retract the needle back into the inserter. During this entire process, pull anterior with the traction suture so the globe is immobilized and there is not a "flick" when the needle disengages from the wall of the globe.

6. Remove the inserter from the eye.

7. Position of the stent in the angle can be confirmed with a goniolens.

8. Test the subconjunctival incision for flow; if present, close with a 10-0 nylon suture.

Postoperative care should include topical antibiotics with frequent topical steroids initially (every 4 to 6 hours while awake) with a slow taper over 4 to 6 weeks depending on the degree of inflammation. Typically, at the 1-week postoperative visit, if the anterior chamber is quiet, the authors begin to taper the steroids down to once a day over the following 3 to 4 weeks. Interestingly, at around the 2- to 3-week visit, one can see a hypertensive phase, and the authors usually begin a timolol drop once in the morning to preemptively treat this phase while continuing to taper the steroids. In terms of needling, the authors will usually treat the IOP with antiglaucoma medications if the IOP increases within the first month. We like to avoid needling within the first 4 to 6 weeks in order to avoid shunting proinflammatory aqueous into the subconjunctival space. Once the eye is quiet and there is no longer any anterior chamber inflammation, one can consider needling. The authors prefer to use the GF microshunt spatula for needling at the slit lamp as well. Depending on the appearance of the conjunctiva around and posterior to the gel stent, the authors will usually augment the needling procedure with MMC (10 to 20 mcg) 10 to 20 minutes prior to the needling procedure.

Grover et al studied the efficacy of Xen through a single-arm, prospective clinical trial.[1] The Xen with an internal lumen size of 45 was used in a standalone procedure, and sponges with MMC were used after opening the conjunctiva. Results showed postoperative IOP at 12 months was reduced 24.7% from preoperative medicated IOP. During the 12 months, 32.3% of patients received supplemental needling of the bleb. The number of medications were also reduced from an average of 3.5 preoperatively to 1.7 postoperatively. In a retrospective study investigating Xen with injection of MMC compared to trabeculectomy with MMC, both groups had similar efficacy of 45.8% reduction of mean IOP; however, there was also no clinically significant difference in complication rates.[2] When investigating Xen with injection of MMC combined with phacoemulsification, postoperative IOP was reduced 41.8% after 1 year without the addition of medications from baseline.[3] Complications can range from subconjunctival hemorrhage, bleb scarring leading to increased IOP, hypotony, choroidal detachment, hyphema, malpositioning, and stent obstruction, to wound leak, conjunctival exposure, blebitis, endophthalmitis, and vision loss. While the side effect profile is not as favorable compared to other angle-based MIGS, its efficacy in patients with refractory glaucoma offers an alternative to traditional filtering glaucoma surgery. As surgeons continue to modify their technique with this device, we will hopefully see improved efficacy with an even lower rate of complications.

PRESERFLO MICROSHUNT

The PreserFlo MicroShunt is an investigational device in final phases of clinical study by the FDA; however, it is being used outside of the United States to treat patients with open-angle glaucoma. The implant is made of bioinert poly(styrene-block-isobutylene-block-styrene), or SIBS. This new and unique compound is flexible enough to mold to the shape of the eye with less inflammation, which leads to less capsule formation.[4] The microshunt is 8.5 mm with an internal lumen size of 70 μm, which at physiologic aqueous fluid production rates should avoid hypotony and IOP less than 5 mm Hg. Migration of the stent is prevented by 2 fins located 4.4 mm from the distal end of the implant. The device is intended to be used in patients with primary open-angle glaucoma who are unable to control IOP on maximum tolerated medications. The surgery can be performed as a standalone procedure or in combination with cataract surgery. Like a traditional trabeculectomy, the implant is used in conjunction with MMC through an ab externo approach; however, unlike trabeculectomy surgery, there is no need to dissect a scleral flap and release sutures during the postoperative period to titrate flow. The luminal diameter and length of the implant limit flow and mitigate the hypotony-related complications that are typically seen with trabeculectomy.

Steps:

1. Using blunt Westcott scissors and conjunctival forceps, create a fornix-based 5- to 6-mm conjunctival peritomy at the superotemporal limbus.

2. Dissect posteriorly and laterally to create a pocket.

3. Achieve hemostasis with bipolar cautery to visualize the scleral bed.

4. Place 3 sponges soaked with MMC (concentration 0.2 to 0.4 mg/mL) into the posterior conjunctival pocket from 2 to 5 minutes (surgeon's preference). Remove the sponges and irrigate the pocket with sterile solution.

5. Mark the sclera 3 mm from the limbus.

6. At this mark, use the knife included in the surgical kit and create a 3-mm long tunnel into the anterior chamber. Downward pressure should be applied to ensure the needle tract is parallel to the iris plane.

7. Use nontoothed forceps to place the **longer** end of the micro-shunt bevel up through the triangular pocket and into the track until the fins on the device are securely snug in the triangular scleral pocket.

8. Confirm proper function of the microshunt by observing drops of aqueous fluid percolating from the distal end of the tube. The proximal end of the tube should be 2 to 3 mm in the anterior chamber. The distal end of the implant should be cannulated with a 25 g cannula and flushed if flow is not initially seen.

9. Bring the Tenon's and conjunctival layers over the implant and close at the limbus using polyglactin sutures to create a watertight seal.

Postoperative care includes topical antibiotics with frequent topical steroids initially (every 2 hours while awake) with a slow taper over 12 weeks.

Currently at time of publication, the PreserFlo MicroShunt FDA clinical trial designed to assess the safety and efficacy of the implant has completed recruitment and is currently under consideration for approval by the FDA; as such, the PreserFlo is not being used currently in the United States. Batlle et al published a prospective single-arm study of Innfocus MicroShunt (Santen Pharmaceutical Co Ltd) in 23 patients in the Dominican Republic.[5] The patients underwent either Innfocus MicroShunt alone (n = 14) or in combination with cataract surgery (n = 9).

Baseline medicated IOP was 23.8 mm Hg, and after 3 years, the mean IOP was reduced 55%. After 3 years, there were no cases of corneal decompensation, late bleb leak, blebitis, endophthalmitis, or vision loss from baseline. One patient required needling of the bleb, and 1 patient required further surgical intervention to control elevated IOP. However, due to the small sample size of the study, these complication rates cannot be applied to the general population. The results from a US clinical trial comparing PreserFlo MicroShunt and trabeculectomy demonstrated a significant decrease in mean IOP and medication dependence in both groups at 12 months. Although the trabeculectomy group had a slightly lower mean IOP on fewer medications, both groups did well with relatively few complications or adverse events.[6] The results from this study were not as favorable as other studies from around the world where high doses of MMC were used. Given the efficacy, ease of use, and favorable side effect profile, the PreserFlo MicroShunt may offer surgeons another promising subconjunctival implant.

CONCLUSION

Over the past decade, there have been several innovations that have provided the ability to create a more controlled and predictable subconjunctival outflow pathway using a microshunt. Both the Xen Gel Stent, as well as the PreserFlo MicroShunt, have been used around the world to safely and effectively lower IOP with a potentially improved safety profile over the standard trabeculectomy in terms of bleb morphology, postoperative recovery, intraoperative safety, and hypotony protection. More data will be required from real-world experience to prove that these microshunts are a significant improvement over the standard trabeculectomy; the authors believe this to be the case, based on the currently available data and personal experience.

REFERENCES

1. Grover DS, Flynn WJ, Bashford KP, et al. Performance and safety of a new ab interno gelatin stent in refractory glaucoma at 12 months. *Am J Ophthalmol*. 2017;183:25-36. doi:10.1016/j.ajo.2017.07.023

2. Schlenker MB, Gulamhusein H, Conrad-Hengerer I, et al. Efficacy, safety, and risk factors for failure of standalone ab interno gelatin microstent implantation versus standalone trabeculectomy. *Ophthalmology*. 2017;124(11):1579-1588. doi:10.1016/j.ophtha.2017.05.004

3. De Gregorio A, Pedrotti E, Russo L, Morselli S. Minimally invasive combined glaucoma and cataract surgery: clinical results of the smallest ab interno gel stent. *Int Ophthalmol*. 2018;38(3):1129-1134. doi:10.1007/s10792-017-0571-x

4. Pinchuk L, Riss I, Batlle JF, et al. The development of a micro-shunt made from poly(styrene-block-isobutylene-block-styrene) to treat glaucoma. *J Biomed Mater Res Part B*. 2017:105(B):211-221.

5. Batlle JF, Fantes F, Riss I, et al. Three-year follow-up of a novel aqueous humor microshunt. *J Glaucoma*. 2016;25(2):e58-e65. doi:10.1097/IJG.0000000000000368

6. Baker ND, Barnebey HS, Moster MR, et al. Ab-externo microshunt versus trabeculectomy in primary open-angle glaucoma: one-year results from a 2-year randomized, multicenter study. *Ophthalmology*. 2021;128(12):1710-1721. doi:10.1016/j.ophtha.2021.05.023

13

Trabeculectomy
Pearls and Pitfalls

Jonathan S. Myers, MD
and Natasha Nayak Kolomeyer, MD

INTRODUCTION

Trabeculectomy remains one of the gold standard surgical procedures for glaucoma. This chapter provides an overview of the procedure and highlights pearls and pitfalls for performing a trabeculectomy. The purpose of trabeculectomy surgery is to create a guarded fistula through which aqueous can drain from the anterior chamber, leading to a steady-state reduced intraocular pressure (IOP). Key steps include scleral flap construction, adjustment of flow through the flap, and watertight conjunctival closure. Excessive fibrosis can lead to bleb failure; therefore, topical steroids and intraoperative antimetabolites (5-fluorouracil or mitomycin C [MMC]) are used to try to prevent fibrosis. MMC is more commonly used and can be applied using a sub-Tenon's injection (see Mitomycin Option #1) or with MMC-soaked pledgets (see Mitomycin Option #2) that are removed after a particular time.

Panarelli JF, ed.
The Pocket Guide to Glaucoma (pp 189-200).
© 2022 Taylor & Francis Group.

Anesthesia

Routine cases can be performed using monitored anesthesia care with intravenous sedation. Additionally topical, subconjunctival, peribulbar, or retrobulbar anesthesia is administered, depending on the patient and surgeon preference.

Superior corneal traction suture is often placed for improved exposure and control. Aim for a longer pass with medium depth.

INJECTION OF MITOMYCIN C (MITOMYCIN OPTION #1)

Inject MMC subconjunctivally as posteriorly as possible (8 to 10 mm from limbus). Use a blunt instrument or cannula to spread the MMC in the bulbar conjunctiva in the planned area of the scleral flap. The absolute dose and concentration can be titrated depending on the patient (usually 0.1 to 0.4 mg/mL; can be diluted with 1% lidocaine). Be careful to keep the MMC away from the limbal edge. It is often more accurate to discuss the amount of MMC used, as opposed to concentration and exposure time.

A superior conjunctival flap can be made one of 2 ways: limbal-based (incision 8 to 10 mm posterior to the limbus; posterior incision) or fornix-based (incision at the limbus; limbal incision). Note that the historical nomenclature is counterintuitive; this can be remembered by noting that the name is related to location of the base or hinge of the conjunctival flap, which is opposite the location of the incision. Incisions at the limbus require less dissection and exposure and may be easier with topical anesthesia. However, these can be more prone to early leaks. Incisions made in the fornix are easier to close and less likely to leak, but they result in a more anteriorly positioned bleb.

SCLERAL FLAP CONSTRUCTION

The scleral flap can be created in different shapes (rectangular, triangular, trapezoidal) and sizes. Prior to incising the flap, it is important to gently cauterize the area to optimize the view, but too much cautery will thin the tissue. The margins of the flap can be outlined at 1/2 to 2/3 scleral depth by using a #67 blade (or equivalent); subsequently a #69 or #57 blade (or equivalent) is used to dissect the flap anteriorly toward the limbus until about 1 mm of the blue-gray zone is exposed. Alternatively, to construct a scleral flap, one can use a bent crescent blade to make a partial thickness groove at the posterior edge of the flap, and then tunnel at that depth forward toward the limbus; Vannas scissors or a blade are subsequently used to cut the sides of the tunnel, creating a flap.

Sutures can be preplaced through the edges or corners of the flap using 10-0 nylon sutures to minimize the duration of uncontrolled flow until the flap sutures are tied down, especially in beginner surgeons.

INSERTION AND REMOVAL OF MITOMYCIN C–SOAKED PLEDGETS (MITOMYCIN OPTION #2)

Avoid mitomycin exposure to the edges of the conjunctival flap. Always count the number of pledgets that are placed and removed. The duration of MMC exposure can be titrated based on likelihood of scarring and/or IOP goal. Wash all MMC from the field before entering the eye in the next step. A paracentesis is placed in a convenient location for postoperative use (usually inferotemporal). The anterior chamber is then entered just posterior to the scleral flap hinge using a sharp blade. A sclerotomy is made with a Kelly punch (Novo Surgical Inc).

A peripheral iridectomy is often performed to prevent occlusion of the sclerotomy with iris tissue, unless the patient has a deep anterior chamber, such as many pseudophakes. However, care should then be taken to avoid a shallow chamber postoperatively, which can predispose to iris incarceration. For the iridectomy, a piece of the iris tissue is grasped with 0.12 forceps with tines parallel to the limbus, to promote a broad-based, rather than long, iridectomy. The tissue is externalized through the sclerotomy and cut using Vannas or iris scissors. The iris is repositioned into the anterior chamber by irrigating with balanced salt solution.

SCLERAL FLAP RESISTANCE

Scleral flap sutures are placed, if they were not already pre-placed prior, and tied down temporarily using slip knots. The resistance across the scleral flap is then tested and adjusted while irrigating the anterior chamber with balanced salt solution through the paracentesis. It is important to note the opening pressure (IOP when flow through scleral flap begins) and closing pressure (IOP when flow through scleral flap stops) and adjust flap tension as needed for the patient. Additional sutures can be placed as needed.

Postoperative adjustment of sutures can allow improved pressure control in the first 4 weeks and may be used to allow a more gradual pressure reduction. Evaluation of the conjunctiva for the likelihood that sutures can be visualized for laser suture lysis (LSL; tissue thickness, risk of subconjunctival hemorrhage) will guide decisions on the use of alternative, external releasable techniques. Several releasable suture techniques are described in an article by Duman et al.[1]

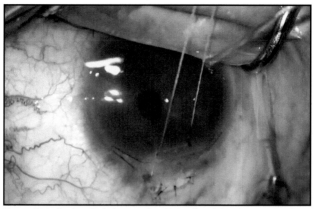

Figure 13-1. Conjunctival closure using 10-0 nylon tight wing sutures. Some choose to place an additional wing suture on each side of the flap.

Conjunctival Closure

Watertight closure is integral to the success of trabeculectomy, as leaks promote bleb flattening and early scarring. There are many different conjunctival closure techniques, some of which are listed below. Commonly used techniques include the 10-0 nylon (nonabsorbable but less inflammatory) and the 8-0 polyglactin (absorbable but more inflammatory).

- Tight 10-0 nylon wing sutures (Figure 13-1) require less manipulation of tissue and needle tracks; however, they require strategic placement of tight sutures. To minimize postoperative astigmatism and unnecessary hooding of tissue beyond the limbus, it is recommended that the sutures are placed close to parallel to the limbus. Often 2 wing sutures are placed, but some choose to place an additional wing suture on each side of the flap.

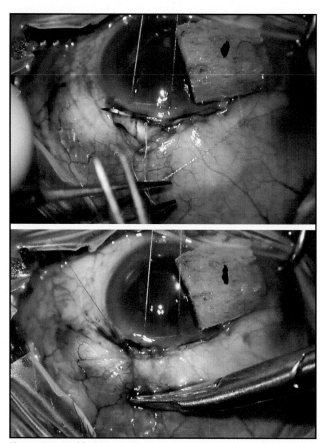

Figure 13-2. Modified Wise trabeculectomy closure using a small conjunctival lip and an 8-0 Vicryl running vertical mattress technique with anchoring sutures at both ends.

- Wise, Modified Wise, or Condon closure (Figure 13-2) using a running vertical mattress technique with anchoring sutures at both ends are described and demonstrated by Kirk and Condon[2]:

- ○ Multiple horizontal mattress sutures
- ○ Running or purse string sutures
- ○ OR a combination of the above techniques

The ideal bleb is shallow, noninjected (but not avascular), diffuse, and may have epithelial microcysts indicating aqueous absorption.

PEARLS/PITFALLS

Patient Selection

Higher risk of failure can be seen in patients with uveitic, neovascular, and aphakic glaucoma, as well as younger patients with thicker conjunctiva, and patients with greater skin pigmentation. Additionally, consider likelihood to attend frequent follow-up and patient cooperation that would be required to perform LSL, digital ocular compression (DOC), releasable suture removal, or needling at the slit lamp.

Optimize Conjunctival Health

It is important to check the health and mobility of the superior conjunctiva. If there is significant toxicity or injection from topical medications, consider stopping them 1 to 2 weeks prior to surgery. Depending on the patient, you can consider adding topical steroids to expedite the recovery of the conjunctiva and/or oral acetazolamide to avoid preoperative IOP spikes.

Minimize Risk of Suprachoroidal Hemorrhage

If IOP is acutely elevated, consider using mannitol or other agents intraoperatively to decrease IOP and minimize the risk of suprachoroidal hemorrhage. Additionally, if the patient is at high risk, you can inject viscoelastic prior to the sclerotomy to minimize acute changes in pressure. The viscoelastic can then be removed prior to tying down the scleral flap sutures to allow more accurate titration of flow.

Know Your Location

Especially for beginning surgeons, it is important to be aware of which clock hour the trabeculectomy flap is being made, as often the traction suture can distort the geography. Some surgeons find it helpful to mark 12:00 or the ideal location of your flap at the beginning of the case. Consistency in placement of the traction suture may aid orientation.

Blunt Dissection

Visualize the tips of your scissors at all times to avoid *perforation of the conjunctiva*. Additionally, always spread and open the scissors, but avoid cutting/closing the scissors in an area you cannot visualize (bluntly dissect as much as possible).

Handling Conjunctiva

Be gentle when handling conjunctival tissue. Avoid use of teethed 0.12 forceps; Hoskins or smooth forceps are more ideal choices. When one needs to place the tissue on significant tension, it is better to **grab Tenon's tissue** rather than conjunctiva itself or grasp the edge of the conjunctiva.

Optimizing the Scleral Flap

It is better to make a thicker/deeper flap outline rather than a thin one, as it gives you more control. Thin flaps can be difficult to close and often result in too much flow. Aim to keep the dissection plane parallel rather than wedge-shaped.

While advancing the flap anteriorly, it is important to not just slide across with a blade. The blade should also have a downward pressure as it is sliding across. Additionally, the opposite hand that is holding up the flap should be pulling up consistently to improve visualization.

If the scleral flap is too thin, you can try to deepen it as you approach the limbus by angling the tip deeper. If flap amputation occurs or you still believe the flap is too thin, suture the flap back down. **It is okay to abandon that site and create a new scleral flap adjacent to this location.** If the scleral flap is deep, avoid involving the vitreous or ciliary body.

Scleral flap sutures that are too tight may be counterproductive, as tissue distortion leads to more leakage. Overriding of tissue can make it difficult to control flow through the opposing area. Tight sutures can also cause significant postoperative astigmatism, especially when closer to the limbus.

Avoid overcauterization, especially at the edges of the scleral flap. This can cause retraction of scleral tissue and eventual difficulties in achieving adequate appositional closure of flaps.

Titrating the Procedure

Before starting surgery, consider your patient's greatest risk. Hypotony? Suprachoroidal? Failure? Prolonged visual recovery in a monocular patient?

Trabeculectomy offers a way to titrate the procedure based on the patient's needs. For example, tight scleral flap sutures would be appropriate in monocular patients or those at high risk for hypotony maculopathy, such as those who are highly myopic. In patients with lower risk of hypotony-related complications, greater flow may increase success. Increased doses of MMC may be appropriate in patients who are at higher risk for scarring or trabeculectomy failure. Wing sutures may be more appropriate in patients with thin conjunctiva that may otherwise tear with running suture techniques. It is important to modify the procedure to fit the patient, while also keeping other parts of the procedure standardized and repeatable, thereby providing consistent but modifiable results. **If you are uncertain, it is better to err toward less MMC and creating a tighter flap.**

POSTOPERATIVE MANAGEMENT
OF TRABECULECTOMY

Digital Ocular Compression

If there is no bleb leak, and the IOP is elevated with a low or flat bleb, DOC can be performed. During DOC, pressure is placed posterior to the bleb to break adhesions and promote flow through the scleral flap interface. This can be performed to **predict** the effect of LSL or to try to **prevent** progressive scarring or early trabeculectomy failure. It should be noted that many types of limbal closure may be at risk of leakage in the early postoperative period (eg, first week) and thus digital compression may need to be deferred.

Laser Suture Lysis

A lens is used to compress over the area of the bleb; the conjunctiva blanches and exposes the scleral flap suture. Argon laser energy is then used to cut the suture and release the tension, potentially increasing flow in that area of the scleral flap. Lenses with focal, convex features (eg, the Ritch and Blumenthal lenses) allow greater compression and visualization of sutures.

Thick tenons or subconjunctival hemorrhage can impede the view and therefore prevent LSL in certain conditions. Hence, some surgeons place external releasable sutures in addition or instead of routine sutures.

Consider noting which flap suture is tighter or more important in determining flow so that you can predict outcomes based on sequence of LSL. As noted previously, you may need to alter the postoperative plan for LSL if visualization is an issue due to thick tenons (cut tighter sutures earlier).

Check the Sclerostomy

If the IOP suddenly increases at a postoperative visit, make sure to check the patency of the sclerostomy using gonioscopy. Iris occlusion of the sclerostomy could be the cause, and pupil distortion may be a clue. This can often be resolved using laser or needling at the slit lamp.

Needling the Bleb

If the sutures have been cut but the bleb remains flat and does not improve with DOC, bleb needling may be indicated.

At the slit lamp, external needling can be performed with the assistance of topical lidocaine gel for anesthesia. Topical phenylephrine drops may also help to decrease bleeding. The goal of needling is to decrease the resistance through the scleral flap and/or above the scleral flap. In the operating room, needling can be performed ab interno and/or externally.

Complications

Complications can include loss of vision, hypotony with or without associated complications (flat anterior chamber, choroidal effusions, hypotony maculopathy, cataract formation, synechiae), elevated IOP, bleb failure, bleb leak, blebitis, early or late bleb-associated endophthalmitis, reoperation, failure, bleb dysesthesia, ptosis, hyphema, vitreous hemorrhage, and suprachoroidal hemorrhage, as well as others.

TRABECULECTOMY-RELATED PAPERS TO FAMILIARIZE YOURSELF WITH

- *MMC Versus 5-Fluorouracil as an Adjunctive Treatment for Trabeculectomy: A Meta-Analysis of Randomized Clinical Trials*[3]

- *Treatment Outcomes in the Tube Versus Trabeculectomy Study After 5 Years of Follow-Up*[4]
- *Treatment Outcomes in the Primary Tube Versus Trabeculectomy Study After 1 Year of Follow-Up*[5]

REFERENCES

1. Duman F, Faria B, Rutnin N, et al. Comparison of 3 different releasable suture techniques in trabeculectomy. *Eur J Ophthalmol*. 2015;26(4):307-314. doi:10.5301/ejo.5000718

2. Kirk TQ, Condon GP. Modified Wise closure of the conjunctival fornix-based trabeculectomy flap. *J Cataract Refract Surg*. 2014;40(3):349-353. doi:10.1016/j.jcrs.2014.01.002

3. Fendi LID, Arruda GV, Scott IU, Paula JS. Mitomycin C versus 5-fluorouracil as an adjunctive treatment for trabeculectomy: a meta-analysis of randomized clinical trials. *Clin Exp Ophthalmol*. 2013;41(8):798-806. doi:10.1111/ceo.12097

4. Gedde SJ, Schiffman JC, Feuer WJ, et al. Treatment outcomes in the Tube Versus Trabeculectomy (TVT) study after five years of follow-up. *Am J Ophthalmol*. 2012;153(5):789-803.e2. doi:10.1016/j.ajo.2011.10.026

5. Gedde SJ, Feuer WJ, Shi W, et al. Treatment outcomes in the Primary Tube Versus Trabeculectomy study after 1 year of follow-up. *Ophthalmology*. 2018;125(5):650-663. doi:10.1016/j.ophtha.2018.02.003

14

Glaucoma Drainage Devices

*Sonal Dangda, MS (Ophthal)
and Steven J. Gedde, MD*

INTRODUCTION

Over the past 2 decades, glaucoma drainage devices (GDDs) have been increasingly utilized in the surgical management of glaucoma.[1] Medicare data demonstrate a 184% increase in GDD surgery between 1995 and 2004 and a concurrent 43% decrease in trabeculectomy procedures.[2] In a recent survey of American Glaucoma Society members, Vinod et al reported that GDD implantation was the preferred surgical approach in 7 of 8 clinical scenarios presented.[1]

INDICATIONS

GDDs have been most commonly utilized in patients with refractory glaucoma (ie, those at high risk for filtration failure):

- Uveitic glaucoma
- Neovascular glaucoma

Panarelli JF, ed.
The Pocket Guide to Glaucoma (pp 201-219).
© 2022 Taylor & Francis Group.

- Traumatic glaucoma
- Fibrous or epithelial downgrowth
- Iridocorneal endothelial syndrome
- Prior penetrating keratoplasty
- Prior retinal surgery (scleral buckling or pars plana vitrectomy)
- Post chemical burn
- Ocular pemphigoid

Recent trends note a shift toward use of GDDs in other ocular conditions[3-8]:

- Eyes without any prior ocular surgery or with previous phacoemulsification (a population at lower risk for failure than has historically had GDD surgery)
- Eyes requiring long-term contact lens use (eg, aphakia, high myopia)
- Eyes that may need additional ocular surgery in the future
- Congenital and juvenile glaucoma
- Concurrent or postkeratoprosthesis placement

CONTRAINDICATIONS

Patients who are unable to comply with postoperative follow-up should be avoided, as GDDs may have a complicated postoperative course. Relative contraindications for anterior chamber placement of a GDD include:

- Anatomically shallow anterior chambers
- Reduced corneal endothelial function

Caution should also be taken in patients with extensive conjunctival scarring where conjunctival closure could be an issue.

MECHANISM OF ACTION

All GDDs consist of a silicone tube extending from the anterior chamber or vitreous cavity to an end plate located in the equatorial region of the globe. A nonadherent capsule forms around the end plate over a period of several weeks after implantation. Aqueous humor pools in the potential space between the end plate and surrounding capsule and passively diffuses through the capsule wall into the periocular capillaries and lymphatics. Primary resistance to aqueous outflow occurs across the fibrous capsule, and the degree of intraocular pressure (IOP) reduction observed is dependent on the capsular thickness and total surface area of encapsulation. In particular, a thinner capsule and larger surface area of encapsulation result in a lower postoperative IOP.[9]

TYPES OF GLAUCOMA DRAINAGE DEVICES

GDDs vary in the size, shape, and material from which the end plate is composed. They are also classified on the basis of presence or absence of a valve. In certain devices, a valve mechanism limits flow through the tube to the end plate when IOP becomes too low. This flow restrictor helps prevent early hypotony. The internal and external diameters of the tube are 0.30 mm and 0.63 mm, respectively. The tube size is similar across the 3 most commonly used devices: Baerveldt Glaucoma Implant (BGI; Johnson & Johnson Vision), Molteno implant (M3; Nova Eye Medical), and Ahmed Glaucoma Valve (AGV; New World Medical). Table 14-1 compares the design and features of currently available GDDs.

Table 14-1. Current Glaucoma Drainage Devices

NAME	YEAR INTRODUCED	MATERIAL	IMPLANT TYPE	SIZE	SALIENT FEATURES
BGI	1990	Silicone (barium impregnated)	Non-valved	250 mm² (103-250) 350 mm² (101-350) Pars plana (102-350)	Both models have fenestrations in the plate that allow for growth of fibrous bands, thereby reducing bleb height The pars plana version has a 90-degree elbow (Hoffman elbow) that aids in tube placement
M3	1979	Polypropylene	Non-valved	**S-Series** 185 mm² 245 mm² (single plate)	Easier implantation due to anteriorly positioned suture holes and a lower profile Unique pressure ridge on the upper surface of the end plate initially limits drainage to small 25 mm² primary area, thereby reducing chances of postoperative hypotony

(continued)

Table 14-1. Current Glaucoma Drainage Devices (continued)

NAME	YEAR INTRODUCED	MATERIAL	IMPLANT TYPE	SIZE	SALIENT FEATURES
AGV	1993	Silicone	Valved	96 mm² (FP8) 184 mm² (FP7; single plate) 364 mm² (FX1; double plate)	Major differences between the FP7 and the older S2 model are the presence of plate fenestrations, a thinner profile, and end plate composed of silicone instead of polypropylene Smaller surface area S3 and FP8 implants are designed for use in the pediatric population

AGV = Ahmed Glaucoma Valve; BGI = Baerveldt Glaucoma Implant; M3 = Molteno implant.

SURGICAL PROCEDURE

Preoperative Assessment

A thorough preoperative assessment is essential. The status and mobility of the conjunctiva and health of the sclera at the anticipated site of implantation should be noted. The presence of peripheral anterior synechiae should be noted on gonioscopic examination if anterior chamber tube placement is planned. A complete ocular motility examination should be performed.

Surgical Technique

Anesthesia

Retrobulbar or peribulbar anesthesia (5 cc) with lidocaine 2% and bupivacaine 0.75% is routinely administered. General anesthesia may be considered in special situations.

Exposure and Dissection

After sterile draping of the operative eye, a lid speculum is inserted. A 7-0 polyglactin corneal traction suture may be used to allow maximum exposure of the selected operative quadrant. The preferred quadrants for implant placement are:

- Superotemporal quadrant: generally preferred, as the surgical exposure is good while postoperative strabismus is less frequent
- Inferonasal quadrant: safe and effective alternative option
- Inferotemporal quadrant: less satisfactory due to presence of inferior oblique muscle fibers and cosmetic issues with the lower eyelid
- Superonasal quadrant: generally avoided, as associated with a higher incidence of diplopia due to the presence of superior oblique muscle and chances of pseudo-Brown's syndrome; additionally, posteriorly positioned implants in this quadrant can potentially encroach on the optic nerve (especially in smaller eyes)

Both limbus-based and fornix-based conjunctival flaps may be used in GDD implantation. The authors prefer a 4:00 fornix-based conjunctival flap along with a radial relaxing incision at each end, as it provides improved exposure. The Tenon's capsule is dissected posteriorly, ideally with blunt Westcott scissors and serrated tissue forceps. The adjacent muscles are carefully identified and hooked. Adequate cautery is applied to the bleeding episcleral vessels.

Priming of Valved Implant

Valved implants need to be primed by irrigating balanced salt solution through the tube with a 30-gauge cannula. This is an **essential step** to open up the valve. In the AGV, priming breaks the surface tension between the valve's 2 silicone sheets.

Attachment of End Plate

The implant may be placed in an antibiotic solution before insertion. The external plate is sutured to the exposed sclera, using 8-0 nonabsorbable sutures (nylon or polypropylene) on a spatulated needle, keeping the anterior border of the implant 9 to 10 mm from the limbus (Figure 14-1). The lateral wings of the 350-mm^2 BGI are tucked under the adjacent rectus muscles while the 250-mm^2 BGI and AGV are positioned between the muscle borders. The suture knots are rotated into the fixation holes to prevent erosion through the conjunctiva.

Tube Occlusion in Non-Valved Implants

As non-valved implants do not have a flow restriction mechanism, temporary occlusion of the tube is required for the first 4 to 6 weeks until fibrous encapsulation of the plate occurs. This may be accomplished in multiple ways.[10-12]

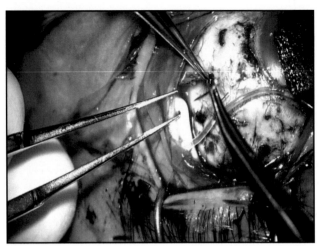

Figure 14-1. The end plate is secured to sclera approximately 9 to 10 mm posterior to the limbus with nonabsorbable sutures (nylon or polypropylene) on a spatulated needle.

External Ligation With/Without Fenestrations

A 7-0 polyglactin suture is externally tied near the tube-plate junction, and complete closure of the tube is confirmed by attempting to irrigate balanced salt solution on a 30-gauge cannula through the tube (Figure 14-2). For IOP control in the early postoperative period, the authors prefer to make a single fenestration anterior to the ligature suture and leave a small portion of a 9-0 or 10-0 monofilament polyglactin suture in the fenestration to serve as a wick-promoting continued aqueous egress (vent and stent technique). Some surgeons prefer to place 1 or multiple fenestrations using the needle on a 7-0 polyglactin suture (TG-140). The 7-0 polyglactin suture ligature absorbs by 4 to 6 weeks postoperatively causing spontaneous opening of the tube. Alternatively, argon laser suture lysis can also be considered depending upon the postoperative course.

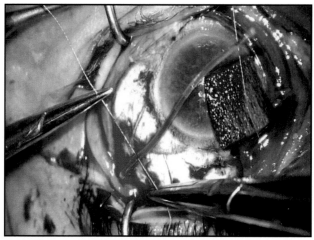

Figure 14-2. Ligating the tube with a 7-0 polyglactin suture near the tube-plate junction restricts flow for the first 4 to 6 weeks after surgery. Complete closure is confirmed by attempting to irrigate balanced salt solution (on a 30-gauge cannula) through the tube.

Ripcord Technique

Ripcord sutures are intraluminal sutures, commonly 4-0 chromic or polypropylene suture. Alternatively, a 4-0 or 5-0 nylon or polypropylene suture is placed alongside the tube and incorporated within the external ligating suture. These ripcord sutures are positioned subconjunctivally in a quadrant away from the implant and can be removed easily after several weeks in the outpatient setting.

Intracameral Suture

Intracameral 9-0 polypropylene suture can also be used. This can be subsequently "melted" with an argon laser to open the tube in office (melt-the-belt technique).

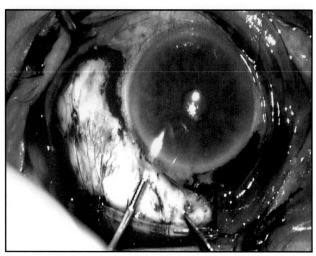

Figure 14-3. After trimming the tube with an anterior bevel, a 23-gauge needle is used to make an entry into the anterior chamber. The tube is inserted through the needle track with nontoothed forceps.

Tube Placement

The tube is cut such that a 2- to 3-mm segment extends into the anterior chamber from the site of entry. To ensure a tight wound, entry into the anterior chamber is made with a 23-gauge needle and the tube is inserted atraumatically with nontoothed forceps. The anterior chamber should be entered parallel to the iris plane, just anterior to the iris insertion, to avoid iris incarceration into the tube opening or corneal contact (Figure 14-3). An anterior tube bevel is made for anterior chamber or pars plana placement, while a posterior bevel is preferred for ciliary sulcus placement to avoid iris plugging the tube opening. Some surgeons prefer to secure the tube to the sclera with a nylon or polyglactin suture.

Tube Coverage With a Patch Graft

The limbal portion of the tube should be covered with a patch graft to decrease the risk of tube exposure over time. The graft can be secured in place with polyglactin sutures. The various options include[13]:

- Partial-thickness autologous scleral flap
- Full-thickness flap/patch
  - Cornea
  - Sclera
  - Pericardium
  - Amniotic membrane
  - Dura
  - Fascia lata

The authors prefer using a human corneal allograft (VisionGraft [CorneaGen]), as it allows for visualization of the ligature if suture lysis needs to be performed and is more cosmetically appealing.

Conjunctival Closure

The conjunctiva is reapproximated up to the limbus and closed with polyglactin sutures (2 running sutures for the relaxing incisions and 1 to 2 horizontal mattress sutures at the limbus).

Depot Medications

A subconjunctival injection (0.5 to 1 cc) of an antibiotic (cephazolin) and corticosteroid (dexamethasone) can be given in the adjacent quadrant. In cases where significant inflammation is anticipated, 0.1 cc of triamcinolone can be injected into the sub-Tenon's space as well.

Postoperative Course

Postoperative follow-up examinations are generally scheduled day 1, week 1, and between weeks 4 to 6 (around the time of external 7-0 polyglactin ligature suture release). Additional visits may be required depending upon the level of IOP and postoperative course.

Topical antibiotic drops are given for 1 postoperative week. Steroid drops to be considered are:

- Prednisolone acetate 1% 4 to 8 times a day for 4 weeks, followed by taper over 2 to 4 weeks
- Difluprednate 0.05% 2 to 4 times a day for 4 weeks, followed by taper over 2 to 4 weeks

The topical steroid therapy may be increased when the tube ligature of the non-valved implant releases, as this event is usually associated with increased inflammation.

Glaucoma medications are generally discontinued in the immediate postoperative period when a valved implant is used or when venting slits/suture wick are used with a non-valved implant.

Occasionally, IOP may become elevated due to the hypertensive phase after ligature release. This occurs as a result of reduced permeability of the bleb, and aqueous suppression can be used to support the IOP during this period. The glaucoma medications can be later reduced, as this condition typically improves with gradual remodeling of the bleb capsule. A hypertensive phase may develop with all types of implants.

Atropine 1% can be considered 2 times a day for 1 to 2 postoperative weeks (especially in cases with a shallow anterior chamber or choroidal effusions) to relax the ciliary body and shift the iris-lens diaphragm posteriorly.

Complications

Complications that may occur during implantation of GDD (intraoperative), within the first few postoperative months (early postoperative) or months/years after the surgery (late postoperative) include[14]:

Intraoperative Complications

- Hyphema (0% to 11%)
- Scleral perforation (0.3%)
- Suprachoroidal hemorrhage (0.5% to 3.5%)
- Vitreous prolapse

Early Postoperative Complications

- Hypotony (3.5% to 37%)
- Choroidal effusion/hemorrhage (7% to 33%)
- Tube obstruction (6% to 11%)
- Aqueous misdirection/malignant glaucoma (0.5% to 2%)
- Wound leak (1.3% to 1.7%)
- Cystoid macular edema/epiretinal membrane (0.3%)
- Decompression retinopathy (1.3%)
- Bleb encapsulation (1.3% to 3.5%)

Late Postoperative Complications

- Erosion/extrusion of the tube or plate (0.5% to 2.3%)
- Migration/retraction of the tube (0.8% to 5.2%)
- Diplopia/ocular motility problem (0.3% to 21%)
- Corneal decompensation (3.5% to 14%)
- Cataract (9.9% to 12%)
- Retinal detachment (3.5% to 5%)
- Endophthalmitis (0.4% to 1.2%)
- Phthisis (1.3% to 4%)

GLAUCOMA DRAINAGE DEVICE OUTCOMES

Glaucoma Drainage Device in Refractory Glaucoma

The type of glaucoma is a major factor influencing the success of any GDD surgery. Eyes with neovascular glaucoma have shown widely variable success rates (22% to 97%) with the GDD procedure.[15-17] When looking at other types of refractory glaucoma, GDD's have success rates of 75% to 100% in patients with uveitic glaucoma, 22% to 58% in eyes post penetrating keratoplasty, and 44% to 100% for developmental glaucoma.[9,18-23] Walton and Katsavounidou noted a 60% success rate for GDDs in eyes with congenital glaucoma, with 62% of these procedures being performed in patients younger than 6 months.[23] Prior to the Tube Versus Trabeculectomy (TVT) Study, various studies noted a 50% to 88% success rate for GDD surgery in aphakic and pseudophakic eyes and 44% to 88% in eyes with failed glaucoma filtering surgery.[9,24]

Comparison of Glaucoma Drainage Device With Trabeculectomy

The TVT Study is a multicenter randomized clinical trial comparing GDDs to trabeculectomy with mitomycin C (MMC). The investigators noted that in patients with prior cataract surgery and/or failed filtering surgery, the success rates were higher in eyes that underwent 350-mm^2 BGI surgery (70.2%) as compared to trabeculectomy with MMC (53.1%) after 5 years of follow-up.[3] The rates of late postoperative complications, serious complications, and vision loss were similar in both groups, while the rate of early complications and reoperation for glaucoma was higher in the trabeculectomy group.[3]

The 2008 American Academy of Ophthalmology update noted level I evidence suggesting comparability of aqueous shunts with trabeculectomy for IOP control and duration of benefit.[25]

Glaucoma Drainage Device as Primary Surgery

The first prospective, randomized trial comparing GDDs to trabeculectomy as primary surgery in low-risk eyes (ie, primary glaucoma eyes without any prior incisional surgery) was conducted by Wilson et al in 2000. They noted a cumulative success rate of 88.1% for AGV and 83.6% for trabeculectomy at 10 months follow-up, and 69.8% in the AGV group and 68.1% in the trabeculectomy group at 3 years.[26,27]

Preliminary results from a more recent multicenter randomized clinical trial, the Primary TVT Study, suggests that trabeculectomy with MMC has greater surgical success and IOP reduction than 350-mm^2 BGI placement in patients who have not undergone previous incisional ocular surgery. However, trabeculectomy with MMC is associated with higher rates of early postoperative complications, serious complications, and reoperation for complications, suggesting a more favorable safety profile for tube shunt surgery over trabeculectomy with MMC in this patient population.[4] Similar observation was reported by Panarelli et al in 125 patients with low-risk glaucoma undergoing primary glaucoma surgery.[5] The cumulative probability of success with or without medical therapy was 87% in the 350-mm^2 BGI group and 76% in the trabeculectomy with MMC group at 3 years. Also, the trabeculectomy with MMC group showed a higher rate of postoperative complications (29% vs 20%) compared to the 350-mm^2 BGI group.

Molteno et al noted a superior IOP control with the M3 as compared to trabeculectomy when used as the primary surgery in 978 primary glaucoma eyes over a period of 30 years.[6] In patients with pseudoexfoliative glaucoma, Valimaki and Ylilehto noted a success rate of 77% at 35 months with the M3 implant.[28]

Comparison of the Various Glaucoma Drainage Devices

The Ahmed Versus Baerveldt Study and Ahmed Baerveldt Comparison Study are multicenter randomized clinical trials comparing the surgical outcomes of valved vs non-valved implants. A pooled analysis of the 2 trials included 514 adult patients with uncontrolled glaucoma that had failed or were at high risk of failing trabeculectomy.[29] At 5 years, the 350-mm^2 BGI group had a lower failure rate (37% vs 49%), lower rate of de novo glaucoma surgery (8% vs 16%), and lower mean IOP on fewer medications than the AGV (FP7 model) group. However, the BGI group carried a higher risk of hypotony (4.5%) relative to the AGV group (0.4%). Prior to that, data regarding the role and efficacy of different glaucoma drainage implant designs were limited to retrospective case series, and most of them used the older poly-propylene (S2) model of the AGV.

Effect of the material or size of GDD on surgical success has also been evaluated in studies. The 350-mm^2 BGI has been noted to have a lower mean IOP compared with the 250-mm^2 BGI implant and a higher success rate than the 500-mm^2 BGI.[30,31] Heuer et al noted a higher success rate with the double-plate M3 as compared to the single-plate implant (71% vs 46%, respectively) at 2 years in aphakic and pseudophakic eyes.[32] However, the risk of postoperative complications due to overfiltration, such as choroidal hemorrhage, flat anterior chamber, phthisis bulbi, and serous choroidal effusions requiring surgical drainage, were also noted to be higher with the double-plate implant. Silicone implants, such as AGV model FP7, have been noted to have a higher rate of success and lower mean IOP than the polypropylene implants, such as AGV model S2.[33,34]

CONCLUSION

GDDs offer a valuable alternative to standard filtering surgery and cyclodestructive therapy in the surgical management of refractory glaucoma. Recent multicenter randomized clinical trials are supporting a trend toward wider use of GDDs in low-risk eyes and as a primary surgical option. Non-valved implants offer better long-term IOP control. Valved implants provide immediate IOP lowering and reduce the risk of hypotony and hypotony-related complications in the early postoperative period. Surgical technique needs to be mastered in order to optimize outcomes.

REFERENCES

1. Vinod K, Gedde SJ, Feuer WJ, et al. Practice preferences for glaucoma surgery: a survey of the American Glaucoma Society. *J Glaucoma*. 2017;26(8):687-693.

2. Ramulu PY, Corcoran KJ, Corcoran SL, Robin AL. Utilization of various glaucoma surgeries and procedures in Medicare beneficiaries from 1995 to 2004. *Ophthalmology*. 2007;114(12):2265-2270.

3. Gedde SJ, Schiffman JC, Feuer WJ, et al. Treatment outcomes in the Tube Versus Trabeculectomy (TVT) study after five years of follow-up. *Am J Ophthalmol*. 2012;153(5):789-803.

4. Gedde SJ, Feuer WJ, Shi W, et al. Treatment outcomes in the primary Tube Versus Trabeculectomy study after 1 year of follow-up. *Ophthalmology*. 2018;125(5):650-663.

5. Panarelli JF, Banitt MR, Gedde SJ, et al. A retrospective comparison of primary Baerveldt implantation versus trabeculectomy with mitomycin C. *Ophthalmology*. 2016;123(4):789-795.

6. Molteno AC, Bevin TH, Herbison P, Husni MA. Long-term results of primary trabeculectomies and Molteno implants for primary open-angle glaucoma. *Arch Ophthalmol*. 2011;129(11):1444-1450.

7. Walton DS, Katsavounidou G. Newborn primary congenital glaucoma: 2005 update. *J Pediatr Ophthalmol Strabismus*. 2005;42:333-341.

8. Netland PA, Terada H, Dohlman CH. Glaucoma associated with keratoprosthesis. *Ophthalmology*. 1998;105(4):751-757.

9. Schwartz KS, Lee RK, Gedde SJ. Glaucoma drainage implants: a critical comparison of types. *Curr Opin Ophthalmol*. 2006;17(2):181-189.

10. Emerick GT, Gedde SJ, Budenz DL. Tube fenestrations in Baerveldt glaucoma implant surgery: 1-year results compared with standard implant surgery. *J Glaucoma*. 2002;11(4):340-346.

11. Yadgarov A, Menezes A, Botwinick A, et al. Suture stenting of a tube fenestration for early intraocular pressure control after Baerveldt glaucoma implant surgery. *J Glaucoma*. 2018;27(3):291-296.

12. An SJ, Wen JC, Quist MS, et al. Scheduled postoperative ripcord removal in Baerveldt 350 implants: a prospective, randomized trial. *J Glaucoma*. 2019;28(2):165-171.

13. Lind JT, Shute TS, Sheybani A. Patch graft materials for glaucoma tube implants. *Curr Opin Ophthalmol*. 2017;28(2):194-198.

14. Lim KS, Allan BD, Lloyd AW, Muir A, Khaw PT. Glaucoma drainage devices; past, present, and future. *Br J Ophthalmol*. 1998;82(9):1083-1089.

15. Sivak-Callcott JA, O'Day DM, Gass JD, Tsai JC. Evidence-based recommendations for the diagnosis and treatment of neovascular glaucoma. *Ophthalmology*. 2001;108(10):1767-1776

16. Assaad MH, Baerveldt G, Rockwood EJ. Glaucoma drainage devices: pros and cons. *Curr Opin Ophthalmol*. 1999;10(2):147-153.

17. Eid TE, Katz LJ, Spaeth GL, Augsburger JJ. Tube-shunt surgery versus neodymium:YAG cyclophotocoagulation in the management of neovascular glaucoma. *Ophthalmology.* 1997;104(10):1692-1700.

18. Broadway DC, Iester M, Schulzer M, Douglas GR. Survival analysis for success of Molteno tube implants. *Br J Ophthalmol.* 2001;85(6):689-695.

19. Coleman AL, Mondino BJ, Wilson MR, Casey R. Clinical experience with the Ahmed glaucoma valve implant in eyes with prior or concurrent penetrating keratoplasties. *Am J Ophthalmol.* 1997;123(1):54-61.

20. Tai MC, Chen YH, Cheng JH, et al. Early Ahmed glaucoma valve implantation after penetrating keratoplasty leads to better outcomes in an Asian population with preexisting glaucoma. *PLoS One.* 2012;7(5):e37867. doi:10.1371/journal.pone.0037867

21. Panda A, Prakash VJ, Dada T, et al. Ahmed glaucoma valve in post-penetrating-keratoplasty glaucoma: a critically evaluated prospective clinical study. *Indian J Ophthalmol.* 2011;59(3):185-189.

22. Budenz DL, Gedde SJ, Brandt JD, et al. Baerveldt glaucoma implant in the management of refractory childhood glaucomas. *Ophthalmology.* 2004;111(12):2204-2210.

23. Walton DS, Katsavounidou G. Newborn primary congenital glaucoma: 2005 update. *J Pediatr Ophthalmol Strabismus.* 2005;42(6):333-341.

24. Hoffman KB, Feldman RM, Budenz DL, et al. Combined cataract extraction and Baerveldt glaucoma drainage implant: indications and outcomes. *Ophthalmology.* 2002;109(10):1916-1920.

25. Minckler DS, Francis BA, Hodapp EA, et al. Aqueous shunts in glaucoma: a report by the American Academy of Ophthalmology. *Ophthalmology.* 2008;115(6):1089-1098.

26. Wilson M, Mendis U, Smith S, Paliwal A. Ahmed glaucoma valve implant vs trabeculectomy in the surgical treatment of glaucoma: a randomized clinical trial. *Am J Ophthalmol.* 2000;130(3):267-273.

27. Wilson M, Mendis U, Paliwal A, Haynatzka V. Long-term follow-up of primary glaucoma surgery with Ahmed glaucoma valve implant versus trabeculectomy. *Am J Ophthalmol.* 2003;136(3):464-470.

28. Valimaki JO, Ylilehto AP. Molteno3 implantation as primary glaucoma surgery. *J Ophthalmol.* 2014;2014:167564. doi:10.1155/2014/167564

29. Christakis PG, Zhang D, Budenz DL, et al. Five-year pooled data analysis of the Ahmed Baerveldt comparison study and the Ahmed versus Baerveldt study. *Am J Ophthalmol.* 2017;176:118-126.

30. Siegner SW, Netland PA, Urban RC Jr, et al. Clinical experience with the Baerveldt glaucoma drainage implant. *Ophthalmology.* 1995;102(9):1298-1307.

31. Britt MT, LaBree LD, Lloyd MA, et al. Randomized clinical trial of the 350-mm² versus the 500-mm² Baerveldt implant: longer term results: is bigger better? *Ophthalmology.* 1999;106(12):2312-2318.

32. Heuer DK, Lloyd MA, Abrams DA, et al. Which is better? One or two? A randomized clinical trial of single-plate versus double-plate Molteno implantation for glaucomas in aphakia and pseudophakia. *Ophthalmology.* 1992;99(10):1512-1519.

33. Hinkle DM, Zurakowski D, Ayyala RS. A comparison of the polypropylene plate Ahmed glaucoma valve to the silicone plate Ahmed glaucoma flexible valve. *Eur J Ophthalmol.* 2007;17(5):696-701.

34. Law SK, Nguyen A, Coleman AL, Caprioli J. Comparison of safety and efficacy between silicone and polypropylene Ahmed glaucoma valves in refractory glaucoma. *Ophthalmology.* 2005;112(9):1514-1520.

15

Childhood Glaucoma
Update on Surgical Management

R. Allan Sharpe, MD
and Lauren S. Blieden, MD

INTRODUCTION

Surgical management of childhood glaucoma depends heavily on the type of glaucoma as well as patient factors, such as age of presentation and medical comorbidities. Traditionally, primary congenital glaucoma is considered a surgical disease with medications employed as a temporizing measure.[1-3] Angle-based surgery, such as goniotomy and trabeculotomy, is widely accepted as the preferred treatment for primary congenital glaucoma, as it has been shown to produce substantial normalization of intraocular pressure (IOP).[2-5] However, careful discernment of the type of glaucoma in the pediatric eye is paramount in selecting the appropriate surgical plan in order to most effectively address the pathology.

Panarelli JF, ed.
The Pocket Guide to Glaucoma (pp 221-234).
© 2022 Taylor & Francis Group.

EXAMINATION UNDER ANESTHESIA

For very young patients or patients that cannot adequately cooperate with an examination in the clinic, it is necessary to perform an examination under anesthesia (EUA). The EUA provides an opportunity for careful examination of the eye, the ability to perform axial length measurements, and photography. Importantly, patients are consented for both an examination and surgery, so that if a surgery is required, it can be done during the same anesthesia event. It is important to discuss with the parents or caregivers that serial EUAs and multiple surgeries are frequently required in the care of pediatric glaucoma. In addition to the risks of the surgeries themselves, there is also a risk associated with multiple exposures to general anesthesia at such young ages.[6]

The standard EUA involves measurement of IOP upon induction of anesthesia, typically prior to placement of an intravenous injection or intubation **if the patient is stable**, to minimize the effect of anesthesia on the IOP. Once general anesthesia is established, measurements of corneal diameter and close inspection of cornea for signs of elevated IOP (eg, corneal edema and Haab's striae) are performed. Retroillumination often helps in visualizing subtle Haab's striae that may not be seen initially on examination with a handheld slit lamp; this needs to be assessed after the patient is dilated. The angle anatomy is then examined with an indirect gonioscopy lens or a direct gonio lens like the Koeppe gonio lens with a handheld slit lamp. The Koeppe provides a great high mag view to appreciate subtle angle structures and postoperative angle changes. The patient is then dilated and a fundus exam is performed with photographic documentation using the RetCam 3 (Natus Medical Incorporated) if available. If not available, a gonio lens can be placed on the eye, and using the center clear lens, one can obtain a view of the optic nerve through a dilated pupil. If one is recording the case, freeze frames can be used to document the optic nerve. In children under 3 years of age, uncontrolled IOP will cause buphthalmos, so ultrasound biometry is performed to measure axial lengths (ALs). The AL of each eye can be compared to age-matched normal values

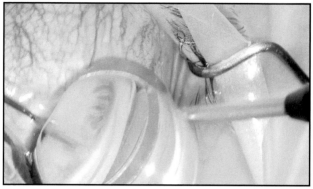

Figure 15-1. Surgical goniotomy cleft.

via plotting on a standardized ocular growth chart.[7] Serial AL measurements are important when following a patient under 3 years old to determine stability of the disease. An asymmetric AL difference between the eyes may be useful in the diagnosis and monitoring of the disease as well. Since the growth of the eye induces axial myopia, retinoscopy can be used to follow these young children as well but is not as precise as AL readings. Asymmetric disease often results in *dense amblyopia*, leading to poor visual development. Monitoring for and treating amblyopia is just as important as treating the disc disease.

SURGICAL APPROACHES

Angle Surgery

Goniotomy

The first angle procedure for congenital glaucoma in the modern era was the goniotomy (Figure 15-1), as developed by Otto Barkan in the 1940s.[8,9] Prior to this, due to the lack of viable treatment options, the visual prognosis for these patients was quite poor with rates of blindness exceeding 80%.[9] His study described the technique of using an *ab interno* approach to incise the trabecular meshwork (TM), and of 17 eyes treated, he reported IOP normalization in 16 (94%).[8] Since then, the reported success rate of goniotomy (either 1 or multiple rounds) falls between 86% to 95%.[10-12]

The goniotomy performed today is remarkably similar to Barkan's description with a few modifications. With the patient under general anesthesia, the eye is prepped and draped in typical fashion for ophthalmic surgery. The surgeon should sit temporal to allow for sufficient access to the nasal angle, although it is possible to perform the procedure in other quadrants or in certain situations. **Remember, a clear cornea is essential for successful goniotomy.** Inspect the cornea carefully before proceeding, as it may exhibit edema or Haab's striae, which can obscure the view. The view of the angle should be confirmed with a sterile, surgical direct gonio lens prior to making the incisions. Some surgeons elect to debride the corneal epithelium or apply glycerin to improve the view with high rates of reported success.[13] In addition, preoperative medical treatment for IOP may be required to reduce corneal edema and ensure a good surgical view. Also, when one makes a paracentesis and the IOP normalizes, the cornea may often clear enough to allow for successful ab interno surgery.

A keratome or 15-degree surgical blade is used to create a temporal clear corneal incision similar to an incision for clear cornea cataract surgery, approximately 2.4 mm in width. The wound should be created with adequate length and distance from limbus to avoid iris prolapse. It is helpful to widen the internal margin of the wound to help achieve a wider arc of treatment. Intracameral preservative-free lidocaine may aid with pain control postoperatively and require less intravenous medication to be given during the procedure. Be aware that intracameral lidocaine may dilate the pupil. A miotic, such as acetylcholine chloride 1:1000 or carbachol, can be injected to constrict the pupil, open the angle, and protect the lens. A cohesive viscoelastic is used to sufficiently deepen the anterior chamber. Depending on the gonio lens used, the microscope may need to be tilted to aid visualization of the angle. The patient's head is often tilted away from the surgeon as well. A surgical gonio lens is then placed on the ocular surface with a viscoelastic coupling agent to visualize the nasal angle. Increased magnification through the operating microscope is critical to adequately view angle structure detail. A 25-gauge 1-inch needle on the viscoelastic syringe is advanced through the corneal wound across the eye with care to avoid catching iris or lens. To avoid injury to the crystalline lens, it is advisable to pass the needle tip over the iris rather than the pupil, if possible. The tip of the needle should engage the anterior TM just posterior to Schwalbe's line. The incision is then extended in a forehand fashion (ie, right to left for a right-handed surgeon) for at least 4 clock hours (120 degrees). The eye and the gonio lens may be rotated to achieve a wider arc of treatment as long as visualization is not compromised. **Successful goniotomy will reveal a widening of the angle, folding over posterior TM, and slow back-bleeding.** Once the incision is complete, remove the needle from the eye and suture the corneal wound with either a 10-0 nylon or 10-0 polyglactin suture. The remaining viscoelastic agent can be irrigated out of the anterior chamber using balanced saline solution. At this point, back-bleeding should be noted from the goniotomy incision. A sub-Tenon's or subconjunctival injection of steroid and antibiotic are given inferiorly (typically triamcinolone 10 mg/mL and cefazolin 100 mg/mL). The postoperative management incudes the use of topical antibiotic and topical steroids. Some surgeons will use either atropine 1% drops or pilocarpine 1% to 2% drops to stabilize the iris and goniotomy cleft during recovery.

Trabeculotomy

In the 1960s, the trabeculotomy was developed simultaneously by Redmond Smith of Moorsfield Eye Hospital and Hermann Burian of the University of Iowa. Smith's technique employed an *ab externo* approach to access Schlemm's canal (SC) and threaded a fine nylon suture. He threaded the nylon several clock hours in one direction then externalized it through another cut down over SC and repeated the same process in the opposite direction. With both tails externalized, he pulled the suture taut, resulting in the

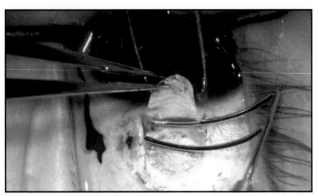

Figure 15-2. Harms trabeculotomes being used in ab externo trabeculotomy. The band of scleral fibers overlying Schlemm's canal is marked with a blue dot.

nylon "burst[ing] through the antero-internal wall of the canal of Schlemm" to create the trabeculotomy.[14] Although Burian's method was similar, he employed a novel device he named the *trabeculotome* (Figure 15-2) and also coined the term *trabeculotomy ab externo* to describe the procedure.[15]

To perform a trabeculotomy, a 3- to 4-hour conjunctival peritomy is created down to bare sclera in either the superior or temporal quadrant. Wet-field bipolar cautery is used to achieve hemostasis. A 15-degree super sharp blade or #67 Beaver blade (Beaver-Visitec International) can be used to create a partial-thickness scleral flap in a triangular or trapezoidal fashion. With the flap elevated, magnification is increased to identify the fibers of SC, which appear as fine, white circumferential fibers just posterior to the limbus. A careful cut down over SC is performed until it is unroofed and aqueous egresses. A corneal paracentesis is made, and a miotic agent and a cohesive viscoelastic are injected.

With the traction suture released, the trabeculotomy can be performed though a variety of methods, such as using the Harms trabeculotome[16] (Rumex Microsurgical Ophthalmic Instruments), 6-0 polypropylene suture,[17] or a fiberoptic lighted catheter.[18] Many prefer using the iTrack 250A (iScience Interventional)

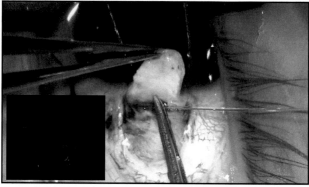

Figure 15-3. Trabeculotomy ab externo using a lighted microcatheter. These stills are taken at the same point during surgery. The inlay shows how dimming the microscope light allows for easy visualization of the red catheter tip as it is progressed through the entire length of Schlemm's canal.

microcatheter when possible, as the lighted tip provides a guide to ensure the device follows the proper course through SC (Figure 15-3). The Harms trabeculotome can be gently placed into the cut end of SC to verify accurate identification of the canal. It is helpful to try to gently rotate the tip of the trabeculotome to confirm placement into SC to encounter slight anterior and posterior resistance. With the trabeculotome removed, the tip of the microcatheter with blinking red light is then introduced into the canal and gently fed through until it circles around fully and is retrieved through the other end. The device should pass smoothly and should not course posteriorly or anteriorly. Each end of the microcatheter is grasped with nontoothed forceps and gently pulled in opposite directions to perform a 360-degree trabeculotomy and completely externalizing the microcatheter.

If the iTrack 250A device does not thread appropriately, the trabeculotomy can be performed with the Harms trabeculotome. Once placed into SC, a slow inward rotation of the trabeculotome should produce little to no resistance upon entering the anterior chamber. The reverse direction can then be treated

Table 15-1. Pros and Cons

	PROS	CONS
GONIOTOMY	No conjunctival manipulation Anatomically precise Less traumatic to adjacent structures Quicker procedure	Requires clear cornea Must identify angle structures Experience with angle surgery required Higher success with primary congenital glaucoma
AB EXTERNO CIRCUMFERENTIAL TRABECULOTOMY	Does not require clear cornea Surgical technique similar to trabeculectomy Ability to treat 360 degrees in 1 sitting	More trauma to adjacent structures Involves conjunctival manipulation Chance of not localizing SC Hypotony possible
SC = Schlemm's canal.		

with the opposite instrument. The Harms trabeculotome set will achieve about 120 to 150 degrees of treatment. Table 15-1 summarizes the considerations when deciding between goniotomy and trabeculotomy.

Gonioscopy-Assisted Transluminal Trabeculotomy and Other Microinvasive Glaucoma Surgery Devices

While not commonly used in the treatment of childhood glaucoma, if the cornea is clear and the view permits, gonioscopy assisted transluminal trabeculotomy may be performed to allow for 360-degree treatment of the TM. However, some groups in the United States and around the world use gonioscopy assisted transluminal trabeculotomy as first-line treatment for primary congenital glaucoma and juvenile open-angle glaucoma.

Currently, in the United States, there are several devices available that may aid the surgeon, such as the OMNI Glaucoma Treatment System (Sight Sciences), the Trabectome (NeoMedix), and the Kahook Dual Blade (New World Medical). At the time of publication, there is no evidence to suggest that any of these devices improve surgical outcomes over simple goniotomy or trabeculotomy in the pediatric glaucoma population.

Tube Shunt

Despite the high success rates of angle surgeries, tube shunt surgery is commonly performed in patients with failed angle surgery or in cases of secondary glaucoma in which angle surgery either has a high likelihood of primary failure or may not be possible. In addition, due to lifelong risks of bleb-associated complications with trabeculectomy, tube shunt surgery is increasingly performed in pediatric patients with refractory glaucoma as an alternative to trabeculectomy. Studies have shown a 70% to 86% success rate with the Baerveldt implant (Johnson & Johnson Vision); however, the use of glaucoma drops postoperatively is common.[19-21] Complications include hypotony, corneal decompensation from tube-cornea touch, implant migration, and tube exposure.[1,21] There is evidence that outcomes are better if a tube shunt is implanted after the age of 3 years, potentially due to fewer tube-related complications from progressive buphthalmos, such as tube movement or malpositioning.[1,22,23] However, if a child requires a tube shunt before the age of 3 years, it is typically because the disease itself is often more aggressive or severe.

Several devices are available to the surgeon. A Baerveldt 350 mm^2 is often used, as these eyes are usually already buphthalmic and can typically accommodate the larger implant. The surgical technique is similar to that employed for adults taking care to ensure that the tube is completely ligated (usually with a 7-0 Vicryl suture) until the capsule has matured around the plate. When there is a high risk of choroidal effusion, such as in Sturge-Weber–associated glaucoma, a staged approach is used where the plate is secured to the globe and the tube tucked back under the plate. Once the capsule has formed around the plate, a second trip to the operating room 6 to 8 weeks later is required to connect the tube into the eye and cover with a patch graft. Alternately, some surgeons employ an *obturator*, also referred to as a *ripcord*.[24] A 3-0 Prolene suture is placed through the lumen of the Baerveldt tube. The tube is then ligated around the Prolene suture using either Vicryl or nylon to ensure that it is watertight at the time of implantation. The other end of the 3-0 Prolene is externalized through conjunctiva during closure. The Prolene can then be pulled out to open the implant in a controlled fashion without a need for extensive dissection. This can be done in the clinic with a cooperative, older child or in a quick return trip to the operating room. The Molteno implant (Nova Eye Medical) is non-valved and has similar considerations as the Baerveldt implant.

The Ahmed glaucoma implant (New World Medical) comes in a smaller pediatric size, Ahmed FP8, but typically the adult size FP7 is employed. The Ahmed implants do not require a ligature and begin to function immediately upon implantation. In general, the Ahmed FP7 device has similar rates of success and complications as the Baerveldt implant[25,26]; however, there is some evidence that Baerveldt produces lower IOP in these patients,[27] and it is left to surgeon preference to determine which implant to use.

Filtering Surgery

Trabeculectomy has historically been employed as the primary alternative to angle surgery prior to the rising popularity of tube shunts, but success rates are variable. Modern techniques using mitomycin C have reported success rates ranging from 39% to 95%, with the mean approximating 70%.[28-33] However, although the use of mitomycin C increases success rates, with it comes increased complication profile, such as hypotony, bleb leak, flat anterior chamber, choroidal effusions, decompression retinopathy, cataract formation, and endophthalmitis.[30-32] There is growing evidence that age of less than 1 year and aphakia portend lower success rates with higher complications.[30,34] The healing response in infants is unpredictable, producing early scarring despite use of antifibrotics in some patients, while hypotony and large avascular blebs develop in others.[1]

Due to the unpredictable nature of trabeculectomy, issues with performing suture lysis, and lifelong risk of bleb-related complications, many surgeons are shifting to employing tube shunts over trabeculectomy in refractory pediatric glaucoma, especially in patients < 1 year old.

Some surgeons are beginning to use microshunts that allow subconjunctival filtration (Xen 45 [Allergan] and InnFocus) in pediatric glaucoma; however, there are very limited data.

CYCLODESTRUCTIVE PROCEDURES

When methods to improve aqueous outflow both medically and surgically fail in pediatric patients, cyclodestructive procedures can be useful to control IOP by reducing aqueous formation.[35] The primary barrier to success is the narrow therapeutic window. The most untoward complication is too much treatment, producing chronic hypotony and ultimately phthisis.[36] Often times, cyclodestructive procedures are most effective after a tube shunt surgery is performed and the eye has a definitive outflow pathway.

To perform cyclophotocoagulation, the Iridex Cyclo G6 glaucoma laser system (Iridex Corp) using the continuous wave G-Probe is used. A total of 14 to 21 spots are placed using 1100 to 1400 mW for 4000 ms. Care is made to avoid the 3:00 and 9:00 positions to avoid damage to ciliary nerves. The power of the treatment should be titrated to the lowest setting. If an audible "pop" is heard, this indicates overtreatment of the ciliary body. The power should be decreased by 50 mW until no pop is heard.

Micropulse laser using the MicroPulse P3 probe (Iridex Corp) is a newer option, with limited data in the pediatric population.

Endocyclophotocoagulation is commonly used in adults with the Endo Optiks microendoscopes (Beaver-Visitec International) and can also be used in the pediatric population. The benefit is direct treatment of the ciliary processes, thereby minimizing total energy delivered and postoperative inflammation. The main disadvantage to endocyclophotocoagulation is that a corneal incision is required and carries the additional risks associated with an intraocular procedure. These methods can be repeated if initial treatment fails to produce desired IOP reduction or effect diminishes over time. However, remember to avoid excessive dosages in retreatment to reduce risk of hypotony.

It is paramount to control inflammation following any cyclodestructive procedure. Some surgeons routinely give subconjunctival dexamethasone and topical atropine at the conclusion of the case and treat with prednisolone acetate 1% 4 times a day for 2 to 4 weeks postoperatively, followed by a weekly taper.

REFERENCES

1. Allingham RR. Medical and Surgical Treatments for Childhood Glaucoma. In: Allingham RR, ed. *Shields' Textbook of Glaucoma*. 5th ed. Lippincott Williams & Wilkins; 2005:626-643.
2. Haas J. Principles and problems of therapy in congenital glaucoma. *Invest Ophthalmol*. 1968;7(2):140-146.
3. Scheie HG. The management of infantile glaucoma. *AMA Arch Ophthalmol*. 1959;62(1):35-54.
4. Scheie HG. Goniopuncture: an evaluation after eleven years. *Arch Ophthalmol*. 1961;65:38-48.
5. Hu M, Wang H, Huang AS, et al. Microcatheter-assisted trabeculotomy for primary congenital glaucoma after failed glaucoma surgeries. *J Glaucoma*. 2019;28(1):1-6.
6. Flick RP, Katusic SK, Colligan RC, et al. Cognitive and behavioral outcomes after early exposure to anesthesia and surgery. *Pediatrics*. 2011;128(5):e1053-e1061.
7. Chang I, Caprioli J, Ou Y. Surgical management of pediatric glaucoma. *Dev Ophthalmol*. 2017;59:165-178.
8. Barkan O. Operation for congenital glaucoma. *Am J Ophthalmology*. 1942;25:552-568.
9. Barkan O. Goniotomy for congenital glaucoma; urgent need for early diagnosis and operation. *J Am Med Assoc*. 1947;133(8):526-533.
10. Russell-Eggitt IM, Rice NS, Jay B, Wyse RK. Relapse following goniotomy for congenital glaucoma due to trabecular dysgenesis. *Eye (Lond)*. 1992;6(Pt 2):197-200.
11. Shaffer RN. Prognosis in primary infantile glaucoma (trabeculodysgenesis). In: Krieglstein GK, Leydhecker W, eds. *Glaucoma Update II*. Springer-Verlag; 1983:185-188.

12. Rice NS. The surgical management of the congenital glaucomas. *Aust J Ophthalmol.* 1977;5:174.

13. Shaarawy TM SM, Hitchings RA, Crowston JG. *Glaucoma: Surgical Management.* Vol 2. 2nd ed. Elsevier; 2015.

14. Smith R. A new technique for opening the canal of Schlemm. Preliminary report. *Br J Ophthalmol.* 1960;44:370-373.

15. Burian HM. A case of Marfan's syndrome with bilateral glaucoma. With description of a new type of operation for developmental glaucoma (trabeculotomy ab externo). *Am J Ophthalmol.* 1960;50:1187-1192.

16. deLuise VP, Anderson DR. Primary infantile glaucoma (congenital glaucoma). *Surv Ophthalmol.* 1983;28(1):1-19.

17. Beck AD, Lynch MG. 360 degrees trabeculotomy for primary congenital glaucoma. *Arch Ophthalmol.* 1995;113(9):1200-1202.

18. Sarkisian SR Jr. An illuminated microcatheter for 360-degree trabeculotomy [corrected] in congenital glaucoma: a retrospective case series. *J AAPOS.* 2010;14(5):412-416.

19. Netland PA, Walton DS. Glaucoma drainage implants in pediatric patients. *Ophthalmic Surg.* 1993;24(11):723-729.

20. Fellenbaum PS, Sidoti PA, Heuer DK, et al. Experience with the baerveldt implant in young patients with complicated glaucomas. *J Glaucoma.* 1995;4(2):91-97.

21. Donahue SP, Keech RV, Munden P, Scott WE. Baerveldt implant surgery in the treatment of advanced childhood glaucoma. *J AAPOS.* 1997;1(1):41-45.

22. Krishna R, Godfrey DG, Budenz DL, et al. Intermediate-term outcomes of 350-mm(2) Baerveldt glaucoma implants. *Ophthalmology.* 2001;108(3):621-626.

23. Chen A, Yu F, Law SK, et al. Valved glaucoma drainage devices in pediatric glaucoma: retrospective long-term outcomes. *JAMA Ophthalmol.* 2015;133(9):1030-1035.

24. Sherwood MB, Smith MF. Prevention of early hypotony associated with Molteno implants by a new occluding stent technique. *Ophthalmology.* 1993;100(1):85-90.

25. Coleman AL, Mondino BJ, Wilson MR, Casey R. Clinical experience with the Ahmed glaucoma valve implant in eyes with prior or concurrent penetrating keratoplasties. *Am J Ophthalmol.* 1997;123(1):54-61.

26. Englert JA, Freedman SF, Cox TA. The Ahmed valve in refractory pediatric glaucoma. *Am J Ophthalmol.* 1999;127(1):34-42.

27. El Gendy NM, Song JC. Long term comparison between single stage Baerveldt and Ahmed glaucoma implants in pediatric glaucoma. *Saudi J Ophthalmol.* 2012;26(3):323-326.

28. Fulcher T, Chan J, Lanigan B, Bowell R, O'Keefe M. Long-term follow up of primary trabeculectomy for infantile glaucoma. *Br J Ophthalmol.* 1996;80(6):499-502.

29. Mandal AK, Walton DS, John T, Jayagandan A. Mitomycin C-augmented trabeculectomy in refractory congenital glaucoma. *Ophthalmology.* 1997;104(6):996-1001; discussion 1002-1003.

30. Freedman SF, McCormick K, Cox TA. Mitomycin C-augumented trabeculectomy with postoperative wound modulation in pediatric glaucoma. *J AAPOS*. 1999;3(2):117-124.

31. Sidoti PA, Belmonte SJ, Liebmann JM, Ritch R. Trabeculectomy with mitomycin-C in the treatment of pediatric glaucomas. *Ophthalmology*. 2000;107(3):422-429.

32. al-Hazmi A, Zwaan J, Awad A, et al. Effectiveness and complications of mitomycin C use during pediatric glaucoma surgery. *Ophthalmology*. 1998;105(10):1915-1920.

33. Agarwal HC, Sood NN, Sihota R, Sanga L, Honavar SG. Mitomycin-C in congenital glaucoma. *Ophthalmic Surg Lasers*. 1997;28(12):979-985.

34. Susanna R, Jr., Oltrogge EW, Carani JC, Nicolela MT. Mitomycin as adjunct chemotherapy with trabeculectomy in congenital and developmental glaucomas. *J Glaucoma*. 1995;4(3):151-157.

35. Bock CJ, Freedman SF, Buckley EG, Shields MB. Transscleral diode laser cyclophotocoagulation for refractory pediatric glaucomas. *J Pediatr Ophthalmol Strabismus*. 1997;34(4):235-239.

36. Hamard P, May F, Quesnot S, Hamard H. [Trans-scleral diode laser cyclophotocoagulation for the treatment of refractory pediatric glaucoma]. *J Fr Ophtalmol*. 2000;23(8):773-780.

16

Landmark Glaucoma Trials

Rachel Lee, MD, MPH
and Kuldev Singh, MD, MPH

INTRODUCTION

Landmark trials are worth close study to understand the basis of current best practices. Here, 7 studies—including the Ocular Hypertension Study (OHTS), Early Manifest Glaucoma Trial, Advanced Glaucoma Intervention Study, Collaborative Initial Glaucoma Treatment Study (CIGTS), Collaborative Normal-Tension Glaucoma Study (CNTGS), Glaucoma Laser Trial, and European Glaucoma Prevention Study—are summarized. This chapter is not meant to be a comprehensive review of the literature but rather a framework to understand the major findings and clinical implications of several key glaucoma trials.

Panarelli JF, ed.
The Pocket Guide to Glaucoma (pp 235-247).
© 2022 Taylor & Francis Group.

OCULAR HYPERTENSION STUDY (2002)

Overview

The OHTS trial was among the first prospective, randomized clinical trials to demonstrate the benefit of treating patients with ocular hypertension to decrease the likelihood of future development of glaucoma. The OHTS trial recruited 1636 participants between the ages of 40 and 80 years, from 22 clinical centers from around the United States. Individuals were randomized into 1 of 2 groups: the treatment group received intraocular pressure (IOP)–lowering topical therapy with a goal of at least 20% IOP reduction from baseline and an IOP of 24 mm Hg or less, and the second group was observed for the duration of the study. All patients had full visual fields and normal-appearing optic nerves on examination (optical coherence tomography was not available at this time). Baseline IOPs were between 24 and 32 mm Hg in 1 eye and between 21 and 32 mm Hg in the fellow eye. One in 4 patients in the OHTS study were Black individuals.[1,2]

At the 5-year mark, the average IOP was reduced by 22.5% in the treatment arm and by 4% in the control arm. Per the original study, ultimately 4.4% of patients in the treatment group and 9.5% of patients in the observation group were eventually diagnosed with glaucoma by the 5-year endpoint.

Multivariable analysis of the original study revealed that predictive factors for the development of glaucoma included older age, higher baseline IOP, low central corneal thickness, higher baseline cup-to-disc ratio, and presence of optic disc hemorrhage. Patients with few or none of these risk factors were found to have low risk of progression to glaucoma (as low as 1% to 2% at 5 years); by contrast, risk of progression was found to be as high as between 25% to 35% of patients in higher risk groups.[1] However, the investigators could not identify a single risk factor that was definitive in predicting the development of early glaucoma.

Several secondary conclusions are worth noting. First, Black individuals were found to be at higher risk for open-angle glaucoma because they were found to have baseline thinner central corneal thickness and larger cup-to-disc ratio. Race was not, however, an independent risk factor for the development of glaucoma in multivariable analysis. Additionally, although the original requirement for diagnosis of glaucoma included reproducible visual field deficits over 2 fields, the investigators found that often these defects would disappear on the third field.[3] Thus, a new diagnosis of glaucoma required 3 abnormal fields. Finally, analysis of the original OHTS cohort over 13 years revealed that optic disc hemorrhages were associated with development of glaucoma. Among patients with disc hemorrhages, the cumulative incidence of primary open-angle glaucoma was 25.6% over 13 years, while those without disc hemorrhages was 12.9%.[4]

Limitations and Criticisms

Patients in high-risk groups as well as those in low-risk groups had comparable IOP-lowering targets. Further research may be needed to determine whether patients in higher risk groups might benefit from a proportionally more aggressive IOP-lowering target. Additionally, less than 10% of patients overall are at risk for progression to glaucoma, and data from the study suggested that time to treatment does not impact outcome; therefore, the decision on when to initiate treatment remains a clinical decision. Finally, the investigators had initially set high standards to make a new diagnosis of glaucoma among their participants. However, through the course of the study, the standards were changed and made even more stringent.

EARLY MANIFEST GLAUCOMA TRIAL (1999)

Overview

The goal of the Early Manifest Glaucoma Trial study was to determine the effect of early, late, or no treatment of patients with **newly diagnosed** glaucoma. The study recruited 255 patients between the ages of 50 and 80 years with newly diagnosed, treatment-naïve glaucoma from population-based screenings in

Sweden. Only patients with mean IOPs lower than 30 mm Hg with neither eye greater than 35 mm Hg were included in this study. Patients were randomized to treatment with either topical beta-blockers or argon laser trabeculoplasty, or observation with or without treatment until signs of progression on 3 reproducible C30-2 fields or progressive optic disc damage, as determined by graders on 3 photographs. Roughly two-thirds of the recruited participants were female, and 1 in 10 participants had pseudo-exfoliative glaucoma. At baseline, the average IOP among study participants was 20.6 mm Hg.[5]

The study revealed that, on average, it takes 4 years from the time of initial diagnosis to the earliest detectable progression of disease.[5] Among those patients found to have visual field progression, the mean median deviation change from baseline was -1.93 dB.[6]

Glaucoma progression was detected in 62% of patients in the observation arm, and in 45% of patients in the initial treatment arm.[5] Overall, the authors concluded that those with at least a 25% decrease in IOP (5 mm Hg, on average) had a 50% decreased risk of visual field progression. Furthermore, each 1 mm Hg decrease in IOP was associated with a lower risk of progression. The protective effect of IOP lowering was present among patients regardless of baseline IOP, age, and stage of disease at time of study entry.[7]

Post-hoc analyses led to several interesting conclusions. First, pseudoexfoliative glaucoma was the only risk factor for increasing IOP over time (roughly a 1–mm Hg increase annually), and also was associated with higher baseline average IOP at enrollment (24 mm Hg as compared to 20 mm Hg among those without pseudoexfoliative glaucoma).[7] Second, a thin central corneal thickness was found to be associated with primary open-angle glaucoma progression, and low blood pressure was associated with progression of normal-tension glaucoma.[8]

Limitations and Criticisms

First, all study participants were recruited from centers in Sweden and, therefore, may not be generalizable to other populations. Furthermore, although the study highlighted the importance of IOP-lowering treatment to reduce the risk of progression of glaucoma, analysis of the data also showed that despite treatment, slightly less than half of patients still progressed. This high rate of glaucoma progression was likely partly due to sensitive criteria to detect progression on visual fields, in which at least 3 test points showed progression on 2 consecutive tests regardless of pattern of visual field deficit. Additionally, it is also possible that IOP-lowering target goals were not aggressive enough, or that there are additional risk factors for progression that remain to be elucidated. Finally, since only argon laser trabeculoplasty and betaxolol were used to lower IOP, generalizability of these results to other forms of IOP-lowering therapies cannot be confirmed.

ADVANCED GLAUCOMA INTERVENTION STUDY (1994)

Overview

The goal of the Advanced Glaucoma Intervention Study study was to determine whether surgical sequence for advanced glaucoma impacts risk of progression. The trial recruited 591 patients (789 eyes) between the ages of 35 and 80 years with advanced open-angle glaucoma with at least 1 eye on maximum-tolerated medical therapy with a combination of persistently elevated IOPs, visual field deterioration, and/or optic nerve deterioration. Patients were randomized to receive either argon laser trabeculoplasty (ALT) followed by 2 trabeculectomies (A-T-T), or trabeculectomy followed by ALT and then an additional trabeculectomy (T-A-T.) Each subsequent treatment step was pursued if a target IOP of 18 mm Hg was not reached in the prior step. Over half of the patients were Black individuals; this subgroup of patients was overall younger and more likely to have vascular risk factors and worse baseline visual field defects as compared to their White counterparts. Patients were followed for at least 8 years.[9]

Overall, the investigators found that average IOPs were lower among patients assigned to the T-A-T sequence. However, subgroup analysis revealed that Black patients—but not White patients—were more likely to progress on the T-A-T sequence as compared to the A-T-T sequence. Visual field defect scores improved among Black patients enrolled in the A-T-T sequence within the first 30 months of follow-up time. Additionally, Black patients were found to be more likely to experience failure with filtration surgery as compared to White patients.[10,11]

Post-hoc analysis of data suggested that patients with advanced glaucoma and average and/or consistently found to have IOPs greater than or equal to 18 mm Hg were more likely to experience progression on visual fields as compared to those who do not.[12] Additionally, patients with diabetes were more likely to experience failure with trabeculectomy.[13]

Limitations and Criticisms

During the first 2 years of study recruitment and enrollment (before 1990), antimetabolites were generally not used for trabeculectomy; however, 5-fluorouracil was used after 1990, and mitomycin C was used after 1991. Because of these changes, the findings of this study are not clearly generalizable to current best practice. The investigators of the study concluded that physicians should recommend ALT, as opposed to trabeculectomy, as a first-line treatment for Black patients with advanced glaucoma. However, close review reveals that all races seemed to require additional intervention if ALT was administered first (30% of Black patients vs 39% of White patients). Similarly, although Black patients were slightly more likely to require additional intervention after a first trabeculectomy, both races were less likely to require additional interventions following trabeculectomy first (18% of Black patients vs 13% of White patients) as compared to ALT first. Furthermore, as this study was conducted during an era in which trabeculectomy surgery was evolving, it is unclear whether or not present-day trabeculectomy with antimetabolites may be better in preventing visual field progression among Black patients as compared to surgeries conducted without the use of antimetabolites in the past.

COLLABORATIVE INITIAL GLAUCOMA TREATMENT STUDY (1999)

Overview

The goal of the CIGTS was to determine whether patients with **newly diagnosed** open-angle glaucoma benefit from early initiation of topical IOP-lowering treatment vs early surgical intervention. The CIGTS trial enrolled 607 patients with a new diagnosis of open-angle glaucoma between the ages of 25 and 75 years of age who had received less than 2 total weeks of IOP-lowering treatment from 11 clinical centers in the United States. Patients were required to have either IOPs of at least 20 mm Hg with reproducible visual field deficits or IOP of 27 mm Hg with optic disc cupping. Patients were then randomized to either 1 of 2 treatment arms: the first group received trabeculectomy with or without 5-fluorouracil, and the second group received a step-wise topical IOP-lowering treatment regimen that was dependent on baseline IOPs and visual field defects. Forty percent of enrollees were Black individuals, 37% of patients had a family history of glaucoma, and average IOPs were 27 mm Hg with a cup-to-disc ratio of about 0.7.[14]

Although patients receiving medical therapy tended to have an initial improvement in visual fields as compared to patients receiving trabeculectomy first, later studies showed that rate of visual field progression were relatively comparable between the 2 groups.[15] Patients randomized to the surgery group had, on average, lower IOP than those in the medication group (between 13 to 14 mm Hg, as compared to 17 to 18 mm Hg).[16]

Post-hoc analyses of data revealed several interesting trends. First, regardless of which group patients were assigned, visual field progression was ultimately detected in between 21% and 25% of all patients.[15] Additionally, 16% of patients receiving initial surgical treatment demonstrated visual field improvement while just under 12% of patients receiving medical management demonstrated improvement in visual field indices after 8 years.

Although, a greater percentage of patients demonstrated visual field loss during the same time period for the 2 groups ($P < .01$ for each).[17] Second, patients with mild to modest visual field defects at the time of enrollment fared equally well in either treatment arm, while those with **more advanced** visual field defects (-10 dB) were less likely to incur visual field progression if they were enrolled in the surgical group.[15] Finally, maximum IOP and IOP range were found to be associated with faster rates of visual field progression in the medically—but not surgically—managed group.[16]

Limitations and Criticisms

The eligibility criteria used to define the study population was broad enough to include some patients who may have had ocular hypertension without perimetric glaucoma. As such, it is difficult to ascertain whether all patients included in the study truly represented patients with glaucoma who would be candidates for filtration surgery.

COLLABORATIVE NORMAL-TENSION GLAUCOMA STUDY (1998)

Overview

The goal of the CNTGS was to determine whether medical or surgical management to lower IOP decreases risk of progression of normal-tension glaucoma. The investigators recruited 140 patients with normal-tension glaucoma, with documented history of progression of glaucomatous disease, or with visual field defects that threatened fixation or new disc hemorrhages. Patients were randomized to receive either medical (excluding beta-blockers and adrenergic agents) or surgical treatment to lower IOP by 30% from baseline, vs no treatment. Overall, the average IOP of the recruited participants was 16 mm Hg. Survival analysis revealed that patients who were observed without treatment for the duration of the study were significantly more likely to progress as compared to patients receiving IOP-lowering therapy (35% vs 12%) and were more likely to do so earlier (4.6 years vs 7.4 years).[18]

Unfortunately, patients in the treatment arm were also more likely to develop cataracts during the study. Thus, due to nonspecific, generalized visual field progression secondary to cataracts, the authors were unable to demonstrate a statistically significant difference in the risk of visual field progression between the 2 groups as a primary endpoint in an original, intention-to-treat analysis. However, after censoring data from patients showing progressive central vision loss due to cataracts, the authors showed that visual field progression is reduced among patients receiving medical and/or surgical IOP-lowering treatment relative to controls who did not receive such treatment.[19]

Limitations and Criticisms

Several shortcomings of the CNTGS included the problems with the initial design and recruitment of patients. Namely, while the investigators called the trial a study of "normal-tension" glaucoma, recruited subjects could have IOPs up to 24 mm Hg, and no central corneal thicknesses were measured or included in the study. Additionally, while prior studies seemed to suggest that disc hemorrhages were associated—but not synonymous—with glaucoma progression, the authors in this study included disc hemorrhages as a potential entry criterion.

GLAUCOMA LASER TRIAL (1990)

Overview

The Glaucoma Laser Trial aimed to determine whether initial topical IOP-lowering medication or laser trabeculoplasty treatment of newly diagnosed open-angle glaucoma was less likely to lead to progression of disease. This multicenter trial recruited 542 eyes of

271 patients in the United States and randomized 1 eye of each patient to receive topical timolol maleate 0.5% twice daily, and the fellow eye to receive argon laser trabeculoplasty.[20]

After 2 years of follow-up, 56% of eyes treated with initial laser trabeculoplasty and 70% of eyes treated with timolol alone required escalation of IOP-lowering therapy.[20] Eyes randomized to receive argon laser trabeculoplasty had better visual field results (0.3 dB higher mean threshold) than those randomized to the topical treatment arm.[21] Long-term follow-up (median 7 years) revealed that patients in the laser treatment arm sustained 1.2 mm Hg greater reduction in IOP, 0.6 dB improvement in visual field, and 0.01 improvement in cup-to-disc ratio, as compared to the topical treatment arm.[22]

Limitations and Criticisms

Because the trial was conducted as a matched-pairs study, data could not be controlled for a small but significant crossover effect of timolol topical therapy on the fellow eye. The possibility of a contralateral effect from laser trabeculoplasty also could not be ruled out.[23]

EUROPEAN GLAUCOMA PREVENTION STUDY (2002)

Overview

The European Glaucoma Prevention Study aimed to determine whether IOP-lowering therapy among patients with ocular hypertension reduced risk of progression to glaucoma relative to a placebo group. In this prospective multicenter trial based in Europe, 1081 patients over the age of 30 years with IOPs between 22 and 29 mm Hg with normal visual fields and optic discs were recruited. Patients were randomized to receive either dorzolamide or placebo eye drops 3 times daily.[24]

After 5 years of follow-up, patients in the treatment (dorzolamide) arm were found to have mean IOP reduced by 22%, while those in the placebo arm had mean IOP that was 19% lower than their baseline. The cumulative probability of demonstrating progression on serial disc photos or visual fields was 13.4% in the treatment arm and 14.1% in the placebo group, which was not a statistically significant difference.[25]

Limitations and Criticisms

Although the study initially recruited a large volume of subjects, the study did ultimately suffer from significant loss to follow-up with over half of the subjects dropping out of the study prior to reaching a final endpoint. Interestingly, the authors also note that patients with higher baseline IOP were more likely to drop out of the study. Thus, although average IOP was found to be lowered to similar degrees in both the treatment and placebo arms, it is possible that this is a result of selective loss to follow-up of the subset of patients with higher IOP, thereby exaggerating the benefit of IOP lowering in both medication and placebo groups.[26,27]

Additionally, because IOP-lowering therapy was not tailored to individual responses to drop treatment and there was no IOP goal established for study participants, it is not surprising that a single medication was not substantially better than placebo.

CONCLUSION

The studies reviewed here influenced best practices in glaucoma. Great care must be taken to interpret and apply these studies in the clinical setting, considering the limitations of each trial, the unique history and circumstance of each patient, and the experience of each physician.

REFERENCES

1. Kass MA, Heuer DK, Higginbotham EJ, et al. The Ocular Hypertension Treatment Study: a randomized trial determines that topical ocular hypotensive medication delays or prevents the onset of primary open-angle glaucoma. *Arch Ophthalmol.* 2002;120:701-713.

2. Gordon MO, Beiser JA, Brandt JD, et al. The Ocular Hypertension Treatment Study: baseline factors that predict the onset of primary open-angle glaucoma. *Arch Ophthalmol.* 2002;120:714-720.

3. Gordon MO, Higginbotham EJ, Heuer DK, et al. Assessment of the impact of an endpoint committee in the Ocular Hypertension Treatment Study. *Am J Ophthalmol.* 2019;199:193-199.

4. Budenz DL, Huecker JB, Gedde SJ, et al. Thirteen-year follow-up of optic disc hemorrhages in the Ocular Hypertension Treatment Study. *Am J Ophthalmol.* 2017;174:126-133.

5. Heijl A, Leske MC, Bengtsson B, et al. Reduction of intraocular pressure and glaucoma progression: results from the Early Manifest Glaucoma Trial. *Arch Ophthalmol.* 2002;120:1268-1279.

6. Heijl A, Leske MC, Bengtsson B, et al. Measuring visual field progression in the Early Manifest Glaucoma Trial. *Acta Ophthalmol Scand.* 2003;83:286-93.

7. Leske MC, Heijl A, Hussein M, et al. Factors for glaucoma progression and the effect of treatment: the Early Manifest Glaucoma Trial. *Arch Ophthalmol.* 2003;121:48-56.

8. Leske MC, Heijl A, Hyman L, et al. Predictors of long-term progression in the Early Manifiest Glaucoma Trial. *Ophthalmology.* 2007;114:1965-1972.

9. Brown RH, Lynch M, Leef D, et al. The Advanced Glaucoma Intervention Study (AGIS): 1. Study design and methods and baseline characteristics of study patients. *Control Clin Trials.* 1994;15(4):299-325.

10. The AGIS Investigators: The Advanced Glaucoma Intervention Study (AGIS): 4. Comparison of treatment outcomes within race. Seven-year results. *Ophthalmology.* 1998;105:1146-64.

11. The AGIS Investigators: The Advanced Glaucoma Intervention Study (AGIS): 9. Comparison of glaucoma outcomes in black and white patients within the treatment groups. *Am J Ophthalmol.* 2001;132:311-320.

12. The AGIS Investigators: The Advanced Glaucoma Intervention Study (AGIS): 7. The relationship between control of intraocular pressure and visual field deterioration. *Am J Ophthalmol.* 2000;130:429-440.

13. The AGIS Investigators: The Advanced Glaucoma Intervention Study (AGIS): 11. Risk factors for failure of trabeculectomy and argon laser trabeculoplasty. *Am J Ophthalmol.* 2002;134:481-498.

14. Musch DC, Lichter PR, Guire KE, Standardi CL. The Collaborative Initial Glaucoma Treatment Study: study design, methods, and baseline characteristics of enrolled patients. *Ophthalmology.* 1999;106(4):653-662.

15. Musch DC, Gillespie BW, Lichter PR, et al. Visual field progression in the Collaborative Initial Glaucoma Treatment Study the impact of treatment and other baseline factors. *Ophthalmology.* 2009;116(2):200-207.

16. Musch DC, Gillespie BW, Niziol LM, et al. Intraocular pressure control and long-term visual field loss in the Collaborative Initial Glaucoma Treatment Study. *Ophthalmology.* 2011;118(9):1766-1773.

17. Musch DC, Gillespie BW, Palmberg PF, et al. Visual field improvement in the Collaborative Initial Glaucoma Treatment Study. *Am J Ophthalmol.* 2015;158:96-104.

18. Collaborative Normal-Tension Glaucoma Study Group. Comparison of glaucomatous progression between untreated patients with normal-tension glaucoma and patients with therapeutically reduced intraocular pressure. *Am J Ophthalmol.* 1998;126:487-497.

19. Collaborative Normal-Tension Glaucoma Study Group. The effectiveness of intraocular pressure reduction in the treatment of normal-tension glaucoma. *Am J Ophthalmol.* 1998;126:498-505.

20. Glaucoma Laser Trial Research Group. The Glaucoma Laser Trial (GLT). 2. Results of argon laser trabeculoplasty versus topical medicines. *Ophthalmology.* 1990;97:1403-1413.

21. Glaucoma Laser Trial Research Group. The Glaucoma Laser Trial (GLT): 6. Treatment group differences in visual field changes. *Am J Ophthalmol.* 1995;120:10-22.

22. The Glaucoma Laser Trial (GLT): 7. Results. Glaucoma Laser Trial Research Group. *Am J Ophthalmol.* 1995;120:718-731.

23. Realini T, Fechtner RD, Atreides SP, Gollance S. The uniocular drug trial and second-eye response to glaucoma medications. *Ophthalmology.* 2004;111:421-426.

24. European Glaucoma Prevention Study (EGPS) Group. The European Glaucoma Prevention Study design and baseline description of the participants. *Ophthalmology.* 2002;109:1612-1621.

25. Miglior S, Zeyen T, Pfeiffer N, et al. Results of the European Glaucoma Prevention Study. *Ophthalmology.* 2005;112(3):366-375.

26. Parrish RK 2nd. The European Glaucoma Prevention Study and the Ocular Hypertension Treatment Study: why do two studies have different results? *Curr Opin Ophthalmol.* 2006;17(2):138-141.

27. Quigley HA. European Glaucoma Prevention Study. *Ophthalmology.* 2005;112:1642-1643.

17

Update on Glaucoma Surgical Trials

Eileen C. Bowden, MD
and Ruth D. Williams, MD

DATA ANALYSIS OF THE AHMED BAERVELDT COMPARISON STUDY AND THE AHMED VERSUS BAERVELDT STUDY

The Ahmed Baerveldt Comparison (ABC) Study and the Ahmed Versus Baerveldt (AVB) Study are 2 independent, randomized clinical trials that compared the Ahmed FP-7 valve implant (New World Medical) to the Baerveldt glaucoma drainage device (350 mm^2; Johnson & Johnson Vision) in patients who were at high risk for filtration failure.[1] The studies were similar in design, patient population, and outcome criteria. Results from the pooled data from these 2 studies were evaluated, offering a greater sample size and greater generalizability than either study alone.

The primary outcome criterion for the pooled analysis studies was failure, defined as intraocular pressure (IOP) > 18 mm Hg or < 6 mm Hg or IOP reduced less than 20% from baseline at 2 consecutive visits after 3 months; repeat glaucoma procedure, such as

Panarelli JF, ed.
The Pocket Guide to Glaucoma (pp 249-259).
© 2022 Taylor & Francis Group.

cyclophotocoagulation or second glaucoma drainage implant (GDI); loss of light perception vision or severe vision loss; and removal of implant.

When comparing the devices at 5 years, the cumulative proportion failing was 49% in the Ahmed group and 37% in the Baerveldt group. The most common reason for failure was elevated IOP in both groups. The cumulative proportion of patients requiring additional glaucoma surgery was 16% in the Ahmed group and 8% in the Baerveldt group.

Both devices were effective in reducing IOP and the need for glaucoma medications. When comparing the 2 groups, the Baerveldt group had a significantly lower mean IOP at all postoperative visits beginning at 6 months and continuing through 5 years. Additionally, the Baerveldt group required significantly fewer glaucoma medications at all postoperative visits, beginning at 6 months and continuing through 5 years. At 5 years, the Baerveldt group had a 2.6 mm Hg lower mean IOP on 0.4 fewer glaucoma medications.

There was a significant reduction in best-corrected Snellen visual acuity that was similar in both groups. At 5 years, 47% of patients in the Ahmed group and 46% of those in the Baerveldt experienced a loss of 2 lines of visual acuity. In the ABC Study, the most frequent causes of vision loss during 5 years of follow-up were glaucoma, retinal disease, and anterior segment pathology.[2] In the AVB Study, the most common cause of vision loss was unable to be determined, but included glaucomatous progression, complications of surgery, and concomitant ocular pathology.[3]

It is important to note that these results may not be generally applicable to the population of patients with no prior ocular surgery. The current Tube Versus Trabeculectomy (TVT) Study seeks to address the question of the role of glaucoma drainage devices as an initial procedure. However, this pooled analysis provides a large sample size, making it useful in comparing the Ahmed and the Baerveldt devices, thereby providing guidance in selecting a device for individual patients.

Ahmed Versus Baerveldt–Ahmed Baerveldt Comparison Expert Opinion

Panos G. Christakis, MD and Iqbal "Ike" K. Ahmed, MD

The AVB Study and the ABC Study provide 5-year, randomized data on the use of these aqueous shunts in patients with refractory glaucoma. While both devices were effective in lowering IOP, there were differences in outcomes that may help guide device selection. The Baerveldt implant achieved a lower IOP on fewer glaucoma medications and should be considered in patients with a low IOP target (< 15 mm Hg) or in patients who are intolerant to or noncompliant with glaucoma medications. However, the Baerveldt implant had higher rates of hypotony and should be used with caution in patients with risk factors for hypotony, including young age and myopia. The Ahmed implant may be a valuable option for patients requiring an immediate reduction in IOP postoperatively. Alternatively, fenestrating a Baerveldt's tube may allow for early flow while the tube is ligated, although the amount of flow may be difficult to predict. Ultimately, selecting a device should balance patient factors with a surgeon's familiarity and personal outcomes with each device.

TUBE VERSUS TRABECULECTOMY STUDY: FIVE YEARS OF FOLLOW-UP

This multicenter, randomized clinical trial compared the safety and efficacy of tube shunt surgery to trabeculectomy with mitomycin C (MMC) in eyes with previous cataract extraction with intraocular lens implantation and/or failed glaucoma surgery. A total of 212 eyes of 212 patients were enrolled, with 107 in the tube group and 105 in the trabeculectomy group. Patients in the tube group underwent placement of a Baerveldt 350 mm^2 GDI superotemporally with complete restriction of flow at the time of implantation. Patients in the trabeculectomy group had a superior trabeculectomy with application of 0.4 mg/mL of MMC for 4 minutes.

Outcome measures included IOP, visual acuity, use of adjunctive medical therapy, surgical complications, visual fields, quality of life, and failure. Failure was defined as IOP > 21 mm Hg or not reduced by 20% below baseline, IOP ≤ 5 mm Hg, reoperation for glaucoma, or loss of light perception vision.

Tube shunt surgery and trabeculectomy both produced a significant and sustained reduction in IOP. At 5 years, IOP was 14.4 ± 6.9 mm Hg in the tube group and 12.6 ± 5.9 mm Hg in the trabeculectomy group (P = .12). Nearly 64% of patients in both groups maintained an IOP ≤ 14 mm Hg at 5 years.

A significantly greater use of adjunctive medical therapy was observed in the tube group compared with the trabeculectomy group during the first 2 postoperative years; however, this difference was not observed at 3 years and all subsequent study visits. The tube group had a higher overall success rate after 5 years.[4]

Treatment failure occurred in 33% of patients in the tube group and 50% of patients in the trabeculectomy group at 5 years (P = .034). The most common cause for failure during 5 years of follow-up in both treatment groups was inadequate IOP reduction. The 5-year cumulative reoperation rate for glaucoma was 9% in the tube group and 29% in the trabeculectomy group (P = .025). There was no significant difference in visual acuity outcomes between the tube and trabeculectomy groups at 5 years.

The results of the TVT study support the expanding use of tube shunt surgery in the management of not only refractory glaucomas but also eyes at lower risk for failure. However, this study does not show either tube shunt or trabeculectomy to be clearly superior to the other. Factors such as surgeon skill, patient-specific considerations, and patient expectations must be considered when selecting the ideal surgical procedure.

PRIMARY TUBE VERSUS TRABECULECTOMY STUDY: ONE YEAR OF FOLLOW-UP

This multicenter, randomized clinical trial compared the safety and efficacy of tube shunt surgery to trabeculectomy with MMC in eyes with no previous incisional surgery. A total of 242 eyes of 242 patients were enrolled, with 125 patients in the tube group and 117 patients in the trabeculectomy group. Patients in the tube group underwent placement of a Baerveldt 350 mm² GDI. Patients in the trabeculectomy group had a superior trabeculectomy with application of 0.4 mg/mL of MMC for 2 minutes.

The primary outcome measure was the cumulative rate of surgical failure at 1 year. Failure was defined as IOP > 21 mm Hg or not reduced by 20% below baseline, IOP ≤ 5 mm Hg, reoperation for glaucoma, or loss of light perception vision.

Treatment failure occurred in 23 patients (20%) in the tube group and in 9 patients (8%) in the trabeculectomy group at 1 year (*P* = .02). The cumulative probability of failure was 17.3% in the tube group and 7.9% in the trabeculectomy group at 1 year (*P* = .01).[5]

The rate of complete success was significantly higher in the trabeculectomy group relative to the tube group (*P* < .001). Inadequate IOP reduction was the most common cause for failure during the first year of follow-up in both treatment groups.

Both surgical procedures produced a significant and sustained reduction in IOP. Placement of a tube produced a 37.5% reduction in IOP, and trabeculectomy with MMC achieved a 46.0% decrease in IOP at 1 year of follow-up. The degree of IOP reduction was significantly greater in the trabeculectomy group compared with the tube group at 1 year. Mean IOP was 13.8 ± 4.1 mm Hg in the tube group and 12.4 ± 4.4 mm Hg in the trabeculectomy group. Mean reduction from baseline was 9.3 ± 6.6 mm Hg in the tube group and 11.4 ± 6.6 mm Hg in the trabeculectomy group (*P* = .02).

Significantly greater use of glaucoma medical therapy was observed in the tube group compared with the trabeculectomy group during the first year of study, though a significant reduction in the use of medical therapy was actually seen in both treatment groups.

The overall incidence of intraoperative complications was similar between the tube and trabeculectomy groups. Early postoperative complications developing within the first postoperative month occurred with significantly greater frequency in the trabeculectomy group compared with the tube group, reported in 20% of patients in the tube group and 33% in the trabeculectomy group ($P = .03$). The rate of reoperation for glaucoma was similar in both treatment groups. No significant differences in visual acuity were seen between the tube and trabeculectomy groups at 1 year of follow-up.

In summary, patients who underwent tube shunt surgery had a higher failure rate compared with those who underwent trabeculectomy with MMC during the **first year** of follow-up in this study. Inadequate IOP reduction was the most common reason for failure in both treatment groups. While trabeculectomy may be a more effective primary surgery, a better safety profile may favor tube shunt surgery. More definitive conclusions can be made when the 3- and 5-year follow-up data become available.

Tube Versus Trabeculectomy and Primary Tube Versus Trabeculectomy Expert Opinion

Steven J. Gedde, MD

The TVT Study found that tube shunt surgery was more likely to achieve surgical success than trabeculectomy with MMC in eyes with prior cataract and/or glaucoma surgery, and both procedures had a similar safety profile. In contrast, preliminary results from the Primary TVT (PTVT) Study showed that primary trabeculectomy with MMC was more effective in providing IOP control than primary tube shunt surgery, although trabeculectomy with MMC was also associated with a higher risk of surgical complications. Results from the TVT and PTVT studies support current practice patterns favoring trabeculectomy with MMC as an initial glaucoma procedure and use of tube shunts in eyes with prior ocular surgery.

There are several limitations to the TVT and PTVT studies that should be kept in mind. Surgical outcomes critically depend on individual patient characteristics, as demonstrated by the different results observed from each trial, and study findings cannot be directly applied to dissimilar patient groups. Although aspects of both surgical procedures were standardized (eg, type of implant, dosage of MMC), some variation in surgical technique occurred because surgeons were allowed latitude to perform the operations in a manner in which they were comfortable. All investigators were proficient in performing both trabeculectomy with MMC and tube shunt implantation. However, many surgeons in practice may have differing experience and skill with each procedure, and this is an important consideration in selecting a glaucoma surgical procedure.

COMPASS TRIAL

The CyPass Micro-Stent (Transcend Medical Inc) is a 6.35-mm fenestrated, flexible microstent with a 300-μm luminal diameter that is inserted into the supraciliary space. It is designed to increase aqueous outflow from the anterior chamber into the supraciliary space via the uveoscleral outflow pathway.

This multicenter, randomized clinical trial evaluated the safety and efficacy of the CyPass Micro-Stent for treating mild-to-moderate primary open-angle glaucoma patients who were simultaneously undergoing cataract surgery.[6] Of 505 participants, 131 patients were intraoperatively randomized into a phacoemulsification-only (control) group and 374 were randomized to a phacoemulsification with supraciliary microstenting (treatment) group.

Outcome measures included percentage of patients achieving ≥ 20% unmedicated diurnal IOP lowering vs baseline, mean IOP change and adjunctive glaucoma medication use, and ocular adverse event incidence through 24 months.

Sixty percent of patients in the control group vs 77% of patients in the treatment group achieved ≥ 20% unmedicated IOP lowering from baseline at 24 months (P = .001). Mean IOP reduction was 7.4 mm Hg for the treatment group vs 5.4 mm Hg for the control group (P < .001); 59% of control patients compared to 85% of treatment patients were medication-free at 24 months. Mean medication use in controls decreased to 0.6 ± 0.8 medications and mean medication use in the treatment group decreased to 0.2 ± 0.6 medications at 24 months (P < .001).

No vision-threatening adverse events related to microstents occurred. There were 8 stent obstructions (2.1%), 2 instances of stent malpositioning, and 2 instances of stent migration or dislodgement. Stent obstructions were related to the formation of focal peripheral anterior synechiae. Greater than 98% of all subjects achieved 20/40 best-corrected visual acuity or better.

This study showed that combining the CyPass Micro-Stent with cataract surgery offers a means to effectively lower IOP and glaucoma medication use in patients with mild-to-moderate primary open-angle glaucoma and comorbid cataracts. **However, review of the 5-year data showed a significant degree of corneal endothelial cell loss in patients with the microstent. As a result, Alcon voluntarily has withdrawn the CyPass Micro-Stent from the market and has asked physicians to cease implantation of the device at the time of this publication.**

COMPASS Trial Expert Opinion

Joseph F. Panarelli, MD

Though the CyPass Micro-Stent is no longer available, the COMPASS trial did provide us with additional important information that is sometimes overlooked. As with other randomized, prospective trials that evaluated canal-based procedures, the control group was phacoemulsification alone. This study once again confirmed that cataract surgery can be an effective procedure at reducing the IOP in patients with open-angle glaucoma. In this study, 60% of controls achieved ≥ 20% unmedicated IOP lowering vs baseline at 24 months. Mean IOP reduction was 5.4 mm Hg in controls with 59% of control patients medication-free. This has definitely impacted my clinical practice, and for most patients who are comfortable with their topical regimen and have controlled IOP, I often recommend cataract surgery alone.

Ab Interno Gelatin Stent in Refractory Glaucoma

The Xen 45 Gel Stent (Allergan PLC) is a 6-mm gelatin tube with a 45-μm inner lumen diameter. A conjunctival peritomy was created during the trial to allow for direct sponge application of MMC to the scleral bed for 2 minutes. The stent was then implanted into the sub-Tenon's space in ab interno fashion via a clear corneal incision under gonioscopic guidance, followed by conjunctival closure.

This prospective, noncomparative, multicenter study involved 65 patients who underwent implantation with the Xen 45 Gel Stent.[7] Primary performance outcomes included patients (%) achieving ≥ 20% IOP reduction from baseline on the same or fewer medications and mean IOP change from baseline at 12 months.

At 12 months, 76.3% patients achieved ≥ 20% mean IOP reduction from baseline using an equal or fewer number of medications. Mean IOP reduction from baseline was 6.4 ± 1.1 mm Hg (95% confidence interval: -8.7, -4.2). Among 52 patients who did not require additional surgical intervention, mean IOP was reduced from a baseline of 25.1 ± 3.7 mm Hg to 15.9 ± 5.2 mm Hg. Mean number of medications decreased from a baseline of 3.5 ± 1.0 (n = 65) to 1.7 ± 1.5 (n = 52).

Postoperative adverse events included transient hypotony (IOP < 6 mm Hg; 24.6%), largely self-limited loss of best-corrected visual acuity > 2 lines (27.7%), and needling (32.3%). One (1.5%) patient developed device erosion requiring surgical revision. Nine (13.8%) patients required additional glaucoma surgery.

This pivotal US Food and Drug Administration (FDA) study of the Xen Gel Stent evaluated a patient population with refractory glaucoma, with the majority having had prior incisional glaucoma surgery. Though the results were encouraging, modifying the technique for implantation as well as MMC use may allow for this device to be used safely and effectively in a broader patient population.

Xen Expert Opinion

Davinder S. Grover, MD, MPH

The Xen 45 Gel Stent is a minimally invasive method for creating subconjunctival filtration. Based on what is currently approved by the FDA, this implant is without question the safest and least invasive method for creating a new outflow pathway in an eye. Subconjunctival fibrosis is still a major battle; however, with the use of MMC, we are able to mitigate the likelihood that the body will completely scar down around this implant. Based on which peer-reviewed paper one evaluates, roughly 20% to 40% of patients require needling in the postoperative period, which can usually be performed safely at the slit lamp. While this implant has not completely eliminated the need for traditional glaucoma surgery, it is a great addition to our surgical armamentarium. I typically depend on this implant in patients who have failed angle surgery or in patients where I do not think angle surgery is likely to work. While Xen 45 was the first microstent approved by the FDA for subconjunctival filtration, it will likely not be the last. My hope is that we will continue to evolve this path of microinvasive filtration surgery and continue to provide our patients safer, more effective, and more predictable surgical methods for the surgical management of glaucoma. The paradigm of filtration glaucoma surgery is rapidly changing, and this is just the beginning of many more exciting things to come.

CONCLUSION

The glaucoma surgical toolkit has grown rapidly in recent decades. The landmark trials included in this chapter have provided important insight into the management of glaucoma and have even influenced shifts in surgical trends. While these data can help guide decision making, each surgeon should assess the individual patient and their individual surgical skill prior to selecting an intervention. Surgeons must also exert caution when applying the results of these trials to dissimilar patient groups. Follow-up data from each of the above trials will provide further valuable information.

REFERENCES

1. Christakis PG, Zhang D, Budenz DL, et al. Five-year pooled data analysis of the Ahmed Baerveldt Comparison Study and the Ahmed Versus Baerveldt Study. *Am J Ophthalmol.* 2017;176:118-126.
2. Budenz DL, Barton K, Gedde SJ, et al. Five-year treatment outcomes in the Ahmed Baerveldt Comparison Study. *Ophthalmology.* 2015;122:308-316.
3. Christakis PG, Kalenak JW, Tsai JC, et al. The Ahmed Versus Baerveldt Study: five-year treatment outcomes. *Ophthalmology.* 2016;123:2093-2102.
4. Gedde SJ, Schiffman JC, Feuer WJ, et al. Treatment outcomes in the tube versus trabeculectomy (TVT) study after five years of follow-up. *Am J Ophthalmol.* 2012;153 (5):789-803.
5. Gedde SJ, Feuer WJ, Shi W, et al. Treatment outcomes in the Primary Tube Versus Trabeculectomy Study after 1 year of follow-up. *Ophthalmology.* 2018;125(5):650-663.
6. Vold S, Ahmed IIK, Craven ER, Mattox C, et al. Two-year COMPASS Trial results: supraciliary microstenting with phacoemulsification in patients with open-angle glaucoma and cataracts. *Ophthalmology.* 2016;123(10):2103-2112.
7. Grover DS, Flynn WJ, Bashford KP, et al. Performance and safety of a new ab interno gelatin stent in refractory glaucoma at 12 months. *Am J Ophthalmol.* 2017;183:25-36.

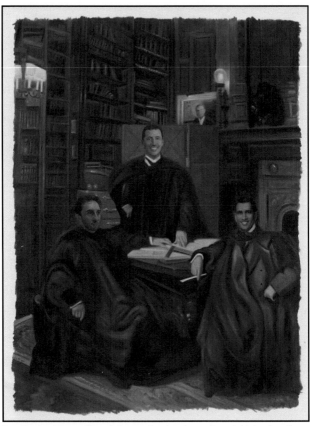

Drs. Sheybani, Panarelli, and Grover planning the outline of this book and pro-
foundly contemplating aqueous outflow.

Financial Disclosures

Dr. Iqbal "Ike" K. Ahmed has not disclosed financial or proprietary interest in the materials presented herein.

Dr. Ahmad A. Aref has no financial or proprietary interest in the materials presented herein.

Dr. Lauren S. Blieden is a consultant for Aerie Pharmaceuticals and Allergan.

Dr. Eileen C. Bowden has no financial or proprietary interest in the materials presented herein.

Dr. Donald L. Budenz has no financial or proprietary interest in the materials presented herein.

Dr. Teresa C. Chen's research is supported in part by the Fidelity Charitable fund.

Dr. Panos G. Christakis has no financial or proprietary interest in the materials presented herein.

Dr. Sara J. Coulon has no financial or proprietary interest in the materials presented herein.

Dr. Sonal Dangda has no financial or proprietary interest in the materials presented herein.

Dr. Anna T. Do has no financial or proprietary interest in the materials presented herein.

Dr. Murray Fingeret is a consultant for Aerie Pharmaceuticals, Alcon, Allergan, Bausch + Lomb, Glaukos Corp, and Novartis.

Dr. Steven J. Gedde has no financial or proprietary interest in the materials presented herein.

Dr. Jeffrey L. Goldberg has no financial or proprietary interest in the materials presented herein.

Dr. Davinder S. Grover is a speaker for Aerie Pharm, Allergan, CorneaGen, New World Medical, Nova Eye Medical, and Reichert; a consultant for Allergan, New World Medical, Nova Eye Medical, Olleyes, RAICO International LLC, Reichert, Sanoculis, and Santen; on the Medical Advisory Board for CATS tonometer, iStar Medical, MicroOptx, and Versant Health; received research funds from Allergan and New World Medical; and received equity from Nova Eye Medical and Olleyes.

Dr. J. Minjy Kang has no financial or proprietary interest in the materials presented herein.

Dr. Janice Kim has no financial or proprietary interest in the materials presented herein.

Dr. Natasha Nayak Kolomeyer is supported by AbbVie, Guardion Health Services, Equinox, Nicox, Olleyes, Santen, Glaukos, Diopsys, and Aerie.

Dr. Rachel Lee has no financial or proprietary interest in the materials presented herein.

Dr. Wen-Shin Lee has no financial or proprietary interest in the materials presented herein.

Dr. Jonathan B. Lin was supported by the National Institutes of Health grants T32 GM07200, UL1 TR002345, and TL1 TR002344.

Dr. John T. Lind has no financial or proprietary interest in the materials presented herein.

Dr. Jonathan S. Myers is supported by AbbVie, Aerie, Avisi, Equinox, Glaukos, Guardian, Haag Streit, MicroOptx, Nicox, Olleyes, and Santen.

Dr. Lilian Nguyen has no financial or proprietary interest in the materials presented herein.

Dr. Joseph F. Panarelli is a consultant for Aerie, Santen, CorneaGen, Glaukos, New World Medical, and AbbVie.

Dr. Ravneet S. Rai has no financial or proprietary interest in the materials presented herein.

Dr. Kitiya Ratanawongphaibul has no financial or proprietary interest in the materials presented herein.

Dr. Joel S. Schuman receives royalties for intellectual property licensed by Massachusetts Institute of Technology and Massachusetts Eye and Ear Infirmary to Zeiss.

Dr. R. Allan Sharpe has no financial or proprietary interest in the materials presented herein.

Dr. Arsham Sheybani is a consultant for Abbvie, Alcon, and Santen.

Dr. Paul A. Sidoti has no financial or proprietary interest in the materials presented herein.

Dr. Kuldev Singh has no financial or proprietary interest in the materials presented herein.

Dr. Kateki Vinod has no financial or proprietary interest in the materials presented herein.

Dr. Jing Wang is a consultant for Allergan and Bausch + Lomb, and received honoraria for Allergan, Ivantis Inc, New World Medical, and Bausch + Lomb.

Dr. Ruth D. Williams has no financial or proprietary interest in the materials presented herein.

Dr. Gadi Wollstein has no financial or proprietary interest in the materials presented herein.

Dr. Eunmee Yook worked with Allergan on the DURYSTA Advisory Board in 2020.

Index

Printed in the United States
by Baker & Taylor Publisher Services